Title: Carb Cycling Cookbook for Sustainable Weight Loss: Unlock the Secret to Effortless Slimming with a 4-Week Meal Plan and Lip-Smacking Recipes for High and Low Carbs Days

Jennifer Napier

Contents

Conclusion **111**

Introduction: The Power of Carb Cycling

Welcome to the journey towards sustainable weight loss and effortless slimming through the power of carb cycling. In this comprehensive guide, we unlock the secret to achieving your fitness goals with a balanced approach to nutrition and meal planning.

We begin by demystifying carb cycling, breaking down its definition and exploring the science that supports its effectiveness in achieving and maintaining weight loss. Beyond shedding pounds, we also uncover the additional benefits that carb cycling offers for overall health and well-being.

Before diving into the meal plans and recipes, we guide you through the process of getting ready for carb cycling. Setting realistic goals, preparing your kitchen, and understanding your body's needs are essential steps in ensuring your success on this journey.

Next, we focus on mastering your macros – the proteins, fats, and carbohydrates that form the foundation of your nutrition. Learn how to calculate your daily needs and adjust your intake accordingly to optimize your results.

The heart of this guide lies in the carb cycling blueprint. Here, you'll find a detailed overview of the 4-week plan, complete with explanations of high carb days, low carb days, and the truth about cheat days.

Packed with mouthwatering recipes tailored for both high carb and low carb days, these dishes will keep your taste buds happy while supporting your weight loss goals.

Finally, we wrap up with a practical guide to meal planning. Follow along with our 4-week meal plan or use the tips and strategies provided to create your own customized approach to carb cycling.

Whether you're just starting out on your weight loss journey or looking for a fresh approach to break through a plateau, the Carb Cycling Cookbook is your ultimate resource for achieving sustainable results and unlocking the secret to effortless slimming. Let's embark on this journey together towards a healthier, happier you.

Let's dive in!

What Is Carb Cycling?

Carb cycling is a dietary strategy that involves alternating between periods of high and low carbohydrate intake. This approach is designed to maximize the benefits of carbohydrates on days when you need more energy, such as during intense workouts, while reducing carb intake on less active days to promote fat loss and improve metabolic flexibility. This method can be customized to fit individual goals, whether for weight loss, muscle gain, or performance enhancement, and requires careful planning of meals and macronutrient distribution throughout the week.

Many people find carb cycling an effective way to lose weight quickly. The initial weight loss is often due to a reduction in water weight, which has contributed to its popularity. Carbohydrates are crucial for providing energy and are measured in calories, similar to proteins and fats. Specifically, carbohydrates and proteins each provide 4 calories per gram, while fats provide 9 calories per gram.

Health authorities generally recommend that daily intake should consist of 50-55% carbohydrates, 10-15% fats, and under 30% proteins. It is important to note that not all carbohydrates are created equal. Healthier carbs come from natural sources such as milk, legumes, whole grains, fruits, and vegetables. In contrast, processed foods often contain added sugars or starches. During digestion, carbohydrates break down into glucose, which the body uses for fuel. Reducing carbohydrate consumption can lead to increased energy levels and decreased cravings.

How Carb Cycling Works?

Taking in carbohydrates results in a rise in blood sugar that, in turn, initiates an enhanced insulin secretion from the pancreas, which subsequently brings the glucose into cells either for energy, storage or conversion into fat however, this process is compensating by the release of glucose into blood circulation (glucagon) when it is needed.

On one hand, high amounts of carb ingest could make your body produce too much insulin. This excess insulin may lead to weight gain and can increase the risk of diseases such as type 2 diabetes and heart disease.

Cycling carbohydrates helps the body restructure its energy system focus on burning fat more than carbohydrates and or muscles as fuel if part of your training you includes exercise and or intense workout for example. Regardless of the lack of long-term studies that illustrate the dangers of carb cycling, it is still deemed an effective dietary approach in short-term application. Maintaining the overall diet is as important as these weight numbers because it is still very effective in managing blood pressure, blood sugar and cholesterol levels.

The Science Behind Carb Cycling and Weight Loss

Carb cycling is a dietary strategy that alternates between periods of high and low carbohydrate intake to optimize energy levels, enhance performance, and promote weight loss. The science behind carb cycling lies in its ability to manipulate insulin levels, glycogen storage, and metabolic flexibility, which collectively support fat loss and muscle maintenance.

Carbohydrates are the body's primary source of energy, and their consumption triggers the release of insulin, a hormone that helps cells absorb glucose from the bloodstream. On high-carb days, increased insulin levels help replenish glycogen stores in muscles and the liver, providing the energy needed for intense workouts and recovery. Conversely, on low-carb days, reduced insulin levels encourage the body to tap into stored fat for energy, thereby promoting fat loss.

Carb cycling can improve metabolic flexibility, which is the body's ability to switch between burning carbohydrates and fats for fuel. By regularly adjusting carbohydrate intake, the body becomes more efficient at utilizing different energy sources. This adaptability can lead to more sustained energy levels, better performance, and a higher rate of fat burning during periods of low carbohydrate intake.

This approach also impacts hormones related to hunger and metabolism. High-carb days can boost levels of leptin, a hormone that regulates hunger and energy balance, potentially reducing appetite and increasing metabolic rate. Low-carb days, on the other hand, help lower insulin and stabilize blood sugar levels, reducing cravings and promoting fat loss.

Carb cycling allows for a personalized dietary plan tailored to individual goals and activity levels. For example, an athlete might consume more carbohydrates on training days to maximize performance and recovery, while someone focused on weight loss might have fewer high-carb days to encourage fat burning. This customization helps individuals maintain a balanced diet without feeling deprived, making it a sustainable long-term strategy.

Implementing carb cycling typically involves careful planning of meals and macronutrient distribution. On high-carb days, the focus is on consuming healthy, complex carbohydrates like whole grains, fruits, and vegetables. On low-carb days, the diet shifts towards higher protein and fat intake to maintain energy levels and muscle mass. This strategic approach helps prevent the negative effects of extreme diets and supports overall health and well-being.

Carb cycling leverages the body's natural metabolic processes to optimize energy usage, enhance performance, and promote weight loss. By carefully managing carbohydrate intake, individuals can achieve their fitness and health goals more effectively.

What Does the Science Say About Carb Cycling?

Regrettably, there is a lack of direct research conducted through Randomized Controlled Trials (RCTs) specifically on carb cycling. The idea of carb cycling draws from other weight loss approaches such as calorie restriction and the ketogenic diet, combined with insights into fueling workouts and fat metabolism. The goal of carb cycling is to synchronize carbohydrate intake with the body's glucose needs.

For instance, prior to longer or intense workouts or races, carb intake is increased (known as "carb loading"). Conversely, on rest days, carb intake is reduced. The rationale behind carb cycling is to adjust carbohydrate consumption based on activity level, reducing carbs on less active days while maintaining protein and fat intake at a steady level or slightly increasing fat intake.

Is Carb Cycling Ketogenic?

Carb-cycling diet and ketogenic diet are obviously not so similar. Whilst the ketogenic diet encourages daily carb intake to be between 20-40 grams to be able to sustain ketosis through period of time when the body utilizes fat for fuel instead of carbs, carb cycling involves fluctuating those levels due to varying carb intake daily. This type of plan cannot be followed at the same time as carb cycling as eating carbohydrates on a ketosis day would cease the ketosis process.

How Many Carbs Do You Need To Lose Weight?

Familiar staples like pasta, bread, rice, and potatoes fall under the category of carbohydrates, often abbreviated as carbs. These are commonly reduced or eliminated when people aim to lose weight. However, carbohydrates are crucial for our bodies as they serve as the primary energy source, particularly for the brain.

Not all carbohydrates are created equal, and understanding this distinction, along with the recommended daily carb intake, can significantly impact health. This knowledge is particularly beneficial for weight management efforts, aiding in both weight loss and maintenance. Registered dietitian Annalise Pratt, RD, LD, emphasizes the importance of striking a balance in carb consumption. Eliminating all carbs isn't advisable as many carb sources also provide essential nutrients like fiber, contributing to overall health and well-being.

How many carbohydrates should you eat to lose weight?

Carbohydrate requirements change due to personal characteristics of age, sex, and activities, thus, most especially during weight reduction. The range of carbohydrate intake as a percentage of the daily calories average between 45%-65%. Taking into the fact that carbohydrates tend to create 4 calories per gram, someone following a 2000 calorie diet need to sticks to a recommended range of 225 to 325 grams of carbohydrates daily.

Effective weight loss involves burning more calories than one consumes. Experts advise aiming for a 500-calorie deficit per day. In terms of carbohydrate intake for weight loss, registered dietitian Annalise Pratt, RD, LD, suggests a range of 100 to 150 grams, which is generally safe for most individuals.

Some may benefit from a consistent distribution of carbs throughout the day. Pratt recommends dividing this into approximately 40 to 50 grams per meal. For instance, a sandwich with two bread slices totals about 30 grams, while adding an apple contributes another 15 grams, totaling around 45 grams of carbs per meal. To manage hunger while meeting carbohydrate goals, Pratt advises incorporating vegetables or healthy fats like nuts into meals.

Calculating how many carbohydrates you need

To ascertain your appropriate carbohydrate intake, utilize the USDA DRI Calculator, a reliable method for gauging your nutrient requirements, especially if you're not following a weight loss regimen, according to Pratt.

Using your height, weight, age, sex, and activity level, the online calculator provides information on:

- Body-Mass-Index.
- On average, daily calorie requirements per day is required.
- Suggested macronutrient intake(nutrients in the forms of carbohydrates, fats, proteins, and fiber)
- Recommended micronutrient intake as well as hydration needs to be indicted.

Do I need more carbs if I'm very active or an athlete?

Individuals who lead active lifestyles and possess greater lean muscle mass can tolerate higher carbohydrate intake levels compared to sedentary individuals. Restricting carbohydrates can negatively impact performance in physical activities or sports, particularly in activities such as weightlifting or sprinting.

National registered dietitian Annalise Pratt, RD, LD, highlights the necessity of providing enough carbs for completion, especially for athletes. Low on the carb stores will give you a great challenge, observed mostly in a marathon. However, the most competitive runners like the bodybuilders use carb cycling and carb loading as a method before the athletic competition to overcome fatigue. Due to limited carbohydrate consumption, the body may need to seek protein as energy instead of using it for tissue repair, rebuilding and rehabilitation.

Are low-carbohydrate diets safe?

Low-carb diets involve limiting the amount of carbohydrates consumed while increasing intake of protein and fats.

According to Pratt, low-carb diets are generally safe for individuals in good health. However, it's essential to maintain a minimum intake of around 130 grams of carbohydrates to support optimal brain and nervous system function. Insufficient carb intake can lead to fatigue and other adverse effects. Additionally, monitoring saturated fat intake is crucial to prevent elevated cholesterol levels.

Pratt advises a balanced approach to weight loss for most people, prioritizing long-term health benefits. This includes consuming carbohydrates moderately and avoiding drastic reductions without medical supervision. If opting for a low-carb diet, Pratt suggests taking a multivitamin to ensure essential vitamin and mineral requirements are met.

Who shouldn't be on a low-carb diet?

Children, pregnant individuals, those highly active in physical activities or sports, and individuals with diabetes should avoid low-carb diets. If you have diabetes, it's essential to consult your healthcare provider before contemplating a low-carb diet.

What are good carbs to eat?

Carbohydrates are categorized into two types, simple and complex, depending on their molecular structure or their form of composition:

1. The simple (or refined) carbs are primarily composed of sugars, and these are less beneficial to the body compared to the complex (fibrous) ones. The group of simple carbs include white bread, potato chips and the cookies.
2. Nutritionally, complex carbs also contain sugars with the advantage that they offer more nutritional benefits such as fiber, protein, vitamins and minerals. Whole wheat bread, oatmeal, and fruits that have undergone a minimal processing are the foods that fall in this category.

Carbs such as whole grains are more satisfying and very effective in keeping one's sugar levels stable.

How do carbohydrates help weight loss?

Making educated decisions regarding your carbohydrate intake can boost your weight loss efforts when paired with a healthy diet and regular physical activity. By reducing overall carb intake and replacing simple carbs with complex carbohydrates and nutritious alternatives, you may improve your weight loss results.

- **Appetite Control:**

Opting for complex carbohydrates, which have a longer digestion process compared to simple carbs, can help you feel satiated and energized for extended periods. This may aid in resisting snacking urges and potentially reducing overall calorie intake. Additionally, the presence of other nutrients like protein or healthy fats in complex carbs contributes to a greater sense of fullness compared to simple carbs.

- **Calorie Burning:**

A study found that adults with a BMI of 25 or higher who followed a high-fat, low-carb diet burned more daily calories compared to individuals following other dietary patterns. This change in metabolism is probably influenced by hormonal responses elicited by dietary choices.

- **Blood Sugar Stability:**

Consuming simple carbohydrates, particularly those high in refined sugar, can lead to rapid spikes in blood sugar levels. To manage blood sugar, consider reducing your intake of simple carbs or replacing them with complex carb options. This approach may aid in stabilizing blood sugar levels and improving overall glucose control.

Healthy sources of carbohydrates

To achieve weight loss or enhance overall well-being, prioritize reducing the consumption of simple and less nutritious carbohydrates such as:

- Sugar-added breakfast cereals or granola bars.
- Candy, sweets, and bakery products.
- Dried fruits, fruit juices, fillers, spreads and jams.
- Snack foods like chips, foods made of refined grains such as crackers, and cookies.
- Sugary fluid like soda, lemonade, energy drink and sports drink are the example of sweeten beverages.
- Sweet starches such as sugar, honey, or maple syrup are sources of calories.
- For example, refined white bread and white rice products.

Instead, aim to incorporate more nutrient-rich complex carbohydrates into your diet, such as:

- They include legumes and beans such as chickpeas, black beans, and lentils.
- High-fiber vegetables including green peas, broccoli, sweet potatoes and butternut squash.
- For example, nuts and seeds can consist of peanuts, almonds, pumpkin seeds, and sunflower seeds.
- Whole fruits like apples and peaches with the rinds still on, all berries that have seeds.
- Whole grains and starches as in rolled oats, barley, whole-wheat bread, brown rice, quinoa or pasta.

Maintaining the weight you lose

Reducing carbohydrate intake for weight loss requires more than just monitoring what you eat. A significant part of the initial weight reduction seen in low-carb diets is due to the loss of water stored with carbohydrates.

To achieve sustainable weight loss, it's essential to combine a balanced diet with regular exercise and address unhealthy behaviors or habits, advises Pratt. Seeking guidance from healthcare professionals such as a nutritionist, registered dietitian, or healthcare provider can offer personalized recommendations tailored to your health status, activity level, and weight loss goals.

Although low-carb diets can result in initial weight loss, achieving and sustaining a calorie deficit often requires more than just reducing carbs, Pratt stresses. Embracing a holistic approach that incorporates diet, physical activity, and behavior modification is essential for long-term weight management and maintaining a healthy weight in the long run.

Benefits of Carb Cycling Beyond Weight Loss

Carb cycling is often celebrated for its weight loss benefits, but its advantages extend far beyond shedding pounds. This dietary strategy can enhance athletic performance, improve metabolic health, support hormonal balance, and contribute to overall well-being.

Enhanced Athletic Performance

One significant benefit of carb cycling is its ability to improve athletic performance. High-carb days ensure that glycogen stores in the muscles are replenished, providing ample energy for intense workouts. This can lead to better endurance, strength, and recovery, making it a valuable strategy for athletes and fitness enthusiasts. By aligning carbohydrate intake with training schedules, individuals can maximize their performance during high-intensity exercise sessions.

Improved Metabolic Health

Carb cycling can also positively impact metabolic health. By alternating between high and low carbohydrate intake, the body becomes more efficient at switching between burning carbs and fats for energy. This metabolic flexibility is crucial for maintaining stable blood sugar levels and can reduce the risk of developing insulin resistance and type 2 diabetes. Additionally, the variation in carb intake helps maintain a healthy metabolism, preventing the slowdown often associated with prolonged low-carb diets.

Hormonal Balance

Another advantage of carb cycling is its effect on hormonal balance. High-carb days can increase leptin levels, a hormone that plays a critical role in regulating hunger and energy balance. Elevated leptin levels can boost metabolic rate and decrease appetite, making it easier to adhere to dietary plans. On low-carb days, reduced insulin levels help stabilize blood sugar, reducing cravings and promoting fat loss. This balance of hormones can contribute to better overall health and mood regulation.

Muscle Preservation

Carb cycling helps preserve muscle mass while promoting fat loss. During low-carb phases, higher protein intake supports muscle maintenance and repair. This is particularly beneficial for individuals aiming to lose weight without sacrificing muscle mass. On high-carb days, the additional carbohydrates aid in muscle recovery and growth, especially after strenuous exercise. This dual approach ensures that muscle tissue is preserved and even enhanced, which is essential for long-term health and fitness.

Enhanced Mental Clarity and Energy

Fluctuating carbohydrate intake can also lead to improved mental clarity and sustained energy levels. Low-carb days can enhance focus and concentration, as the body efficiently burns fat for fuel, which provides a steady energy supply. Conversely, high-carb days can boost energy levels and mood, particularly when timed around physical activity. This balance helps maintain cognitive function and overall energy throughout the week.

Sustainable Eating Habits

Finally, carb cycling promotes sustainable eating habits. The flexibility of this approach allows individuals to enjoy a variety of foods without feeling deprived. By incorporating both high and low-carb days, people can indulge in their favorite carbohydrate-rich foods in moderation, reducing the likelihood of binge eating and improving adherence to long-term dietary goals. This balance fosters a healthier relationship with food and encourages mindful eating practices.

Carb cycling offers numerous benefits beyond weight loss, including enhanced athletic performance, improved metabolic health, hormonal balance, muscle preservation, mental clarity, and sustainable eating habits. By strategically varying carbohydrate intake, individuals can achieve a comprehensive approach to health and fitness.

Few drawbacks of Carb Cycling

May Go Overboard with Carbs

The implementation of a carb cycling diet can pose challenges, leading some to argue that it's more suitable for elite endurance athletes rather than individuals aiming for weight loss. The complexity arises from determining the appropriate carbohydrate intake levels for low, moderate, and high carbohydrate days.

For instance, on low-carb days, one might consume roughly 2 ½ to 5 servings of carbohydrate-rich foods, while high-carb days may involve 10 to 20 servings. Furthermore, the diet requires meticulous tracking of carbohydrates, protein, and fat, making it time-consuming. Without careful monitoring of carb intake, there's a risk of deviating from the intended dietary plan.

May Develop an Unhealthy Relationship with Food

While short-term adherence to carb cycling is feasible, maintaining this dietary approach long-term can pose challenges. Similar to other restrictive diets, there's a potential risk of developing an unhealthy fixation on healthy eating, referred to as orthorexia.

 On low-carb days, cravings for high-carb foods may persist, possibly leading to binge eating on high-carb days. Moreover, carb cycling overlooks individual appetite variations. Some individuals experience reduced appetite on intense training days compared to rest days, making it unsustainable to follow a super-low-carb regimen when appetite is high.

It's Not Safe for Certain People

Carb cycling isn't advised for individuals with diabetes or low blood sugar, as they need a consistent glucose supply. Additionally, restricting nutrient-rich carb sources, like fortified grains, could lead to health issues. This is particularly concerning for women of childbearing age, who often have low iron and folic acid levels. Inadequate fiber intake from limiting carb-rich foods may also cause constipation.

Must Read!!!

Thank you for choosing to explore my book! Your support means the world to me. As a valued reader, your review holds immense significance. Your insights not only guide potential readers but also contribute to shaping the ongoing journey of this book. Your thoughts help in fostering a community of engaged readers, making the experience richer for everyone.

How You Can Share Your Review?

Sharing your review on Amazon allows others to benefit from your perspective, aiding them in their decision-making process.

To post your review, simply visit the Amazon page where you discovered my book, head to the 'Customer Reviews' section, and click on 'Write a customer review' to share your invaluable feedback.

Alternatively, you can effortlessly access the review section by scanning the QR code below with your smartphone. Thank you once again for your support and for considering sharing your thoughts with us.

Chapter 2: Getting Ready for Carb Cycling

Setting Realistic Goals for Carb Cycling

Carb cycling can be an effective dietary strategy for achieving various health and fitness objectives. Setting realistic goals is crucial for maximizing the benefits and maintaining long-term adherence. One of the primary goals of carb cycling is weight loss. By alternating between high and low carbohydrate days, you can create a calorie deficit while maintaining energy levels for workouts.

A realistic weight loss goal is to aim for a gradual reduction of 1-2 pounds per week, which helps ensure fat loss rather than muscle loss and supports long-term success. For those looking to build or preserve muscle, carb cycling can be particularly beneficial. High-carb days can support intense strength training sessions by providing the necessary energy and aiding in muscle recovery and growth. A realistic goal is to aim for a gradual increase in muscle mass, around 0.5-1 pound per month, depending on your training intensity and consistency.

Enhancing athletic performance is another realistic goal with carb cycling. By timing high-carb days around intense training sessions or competitions, you can ensure that glycogen stores are replenished, leading to better performance and faster recovery.

A realistic goal is to improve your performance metrics, such as running speed, lifting capacity, or endurance, incrementally over several months. Improving metabolic health is a long-term goal that can be achieved through carb cycling. By increasing metabolic flexibility and improving insulin sensitivity, you can reduce the risk of metabolic diseases. A realistic goal is to see improvements in blood sugar levels, cholesterol profiles, and body composition over a period of three to six months.

Carb cycling can help stabilize energy levels and improve mental clarity by preventing the energy crashes often associated with high-carb diets. A realistic goal is to achieve more consistent energy throughout the day and enhanced cognitive function, noticeable within a few weeks of starting the carb cycling regimen.

Achieving hormonal balance is a significant benefit of carb cycling, particularly for regulating hunger hormones like leptin and insulin. A realistic goal is to experience reduced cravings and more stable appetite control within a month. For women, it can also mean more regular menstrual cycles and reduced symptoms of hormonal imbalances over several months.

Developing sustainable eating habits is a critical goal for long-term health. Carb cycling allows for flexibility in your diet, helping you to avoid feelings of deprivation. A realistic goal is to establish a balanced and varied eating pattern that you can maintain comfortably for six months to a year and beyond.

Improving body composition involves reducing body fat while maintaining or increasing muscle mass. With carb cycling, a realistic goal is to see a gradual improvement in body composition over a three to six-month period. This can be measured by tracking changes in body fat percentage and muscle mass through methods such as bioelectrical impedance analysis or DEXA scans.

For those engaged in regular physical activity, improved recovery and reduced inflammation are important goals. Carb cycling can help manage inflammation by balancing carbohydrate intake with periods of lower carb consumption.

A realistic goal is to notice reduced muscle soreness and quicker recovery times within a few weeks of implementing carb cycling. Finally, developing a healthier relationship with food is a crucial goal. Carb cycling encourages mindful eating and a better understanding of how different foods impact your body. A realistic goal is to feel more in control of your eating habits and experience less guilt or stress related to food within a few months.

Carb cycling can support a variety of realistic health and fitness goals, including weight loss, muscle gain, improved performance, enhanced metabolic health, better energy levels, hormonal balance, sustainable eating habits, improved body composition, reduced inflammation, and a healthier relationship with food. Setting specific, measurable, and achievable goals can help you maximize the benefits of carb cycling and maintain long-term success.

Carb Cycle Meal Plan

Within the dynamic realm of health and fitness, where dietary trends come and go, carb cycling is a flexible method that is gaining traction with people looking for a sustainable and well-rounded nutritional plan. Carb cycling is a particularly useful strategy for addressing the dynamic nature of our energy demands while also accommodating a variety of lifestyles, particularly as we traverse the complexity of contemporary nutritional options.

What Is a Carb Cycling Schedule?

Fundamentally, carb cycling is a deliberate ebb and flow in the amount of carbohydrates consumed, resulting in a cyclic pattern that corresponds with varying degrees of activity. The idea is basic but effective: we want to maximize energy use and metabolic efficiency by timing our intake of carbohydrates with our daily activities. In an effort to help you make sense of the complex world of carb cycling, this guide will walk you through its definition, explain the science underlying its benefits, and help you decide if it is a good fit for your own fitness and health goals.

We will go through the essentials of carb cycling as we set out on this journey, illuminating both its advantages and its disadvantages. We want to provide you with the information you need to make thoughtful and significant decisions about your nutritional strategy, from knowing when to use a carb cycling method to creating a meal plan specific to your training schedule.

Carb cycling is a strategic approach to nutrition that acknowledges the dynamic nature of our bodies' energy requirements. It is not merely a diet. Fundamentally, carb cycling is the intentional control of the amount of carbohydrates consumed, with intervals of increased and decreased consumption spread out over the course of the week or month. The secret is to align these oscillations with your exercise needs in order to maximize energy, performance, and metabolic reactions.

Understanding the function of carbs in our bodies is crucial to understanding the fundamentals of carb cycling. The main source of energy for many physiological functions is glucose. Still, not every day is created equal when it comes to energy use. To maintain optimal performance and replace glycogen reserves, your body may benefit from a larger intake of carbs on days of strong physical activity or strenuous training. On the other hand, consuming fewer carbohydrates could encourage the body to use fat reserves as an energy source on days when you are not as active or spend more time sleeping.

This approach's cyclical structure provides flexibility, enabling it to be tailored to a range of lifestyles and fitness objectives. It is a customized method that can be adjusted to suit specific requirements and preferences rather than a one-size-fits-all approach. While some would choose a longer pattern, varying their carbohydrate consumption over the course of a month, others might choose a weekly cycle with high and low-carb days.

When is a Meal Plan for Carb Cycling Appropriate?

In some fitness scenarios, where its adjustable nature matches individual goals, carb cycling proved useful. It is especially helpful for those who work out at different intensities since it adjusts carbohydrate intake to suit different degrees of exercise, improving both performance and recovery. This method offers a balanced strategy for fat reduction while maintaining lean muscle mass, making it suitable for people who are trying to achieve goals related to body composition.

By matching their carbohydrate intake to high-intensity training sessions, endurance athletes can benefit from carb cycling, which promotes sustained energy during extended activities. Carb cycling provides sporadic higher-carb days to people battling diet-induced tiredness on long-term low-carb regimens, refueling glycogen reserves and promoting sustainable energy levels.

Despite its advantages, carb cycling adoption is a personal decision influenced by dietary preferences, individual sensitivities, and general health concerns. Consulting with healthcare experts guarantees a customized strategy that fits each person's requirements and situation.

Preparing Your Kitchen for Success

Preparing your kitchen for success with carb cycling involves stocking up on the right ingredients and organizing your space to make meal prep easier. Here's a guide to get you started:

Understand Carb Cycling: Before you start prepping your kitchen, make sure you understand the principles of carb cycling. It involves alternating between high-carb days, low-carb days, and sometimes no-carb days to manipulate your body's fuel sources and promote fat loss while preserving muscle mass.

Plan Your Meals: Based on your carb cycling plan, create a weekly meal plan. This will help you know exactly what ingredients you need and when to use them.

Stock Up on the Basics:

- High-Carb Days: Whole grains like brown rice, quinoa, oats; starchy vegetables like sweet potatoes, corn, peas; fruits like bananas, berries, apples.
- Low-Carb Days: Lean proteins such as chicken, turkey, fish, tofu; non-starchy vegetables like spinach, broccoli, cauliflower; healthy fats like avocados, nuts, olive oil.
- No-Carb Days (if applicable): Focus on lean proteins, non-starchy vegetables, and healthy fats.

Organize Your Kitchen:

- Keep high-carb and low-carb ingredients separate and easily accessible.
- Use clear containers for pantry staples like rice, quinoa, and oats for easy visibility.
- Store fruits and vegetables in the fridge in designated bins to keep them fresh.

Keep healthy snacks like nuts and seeds in portioned containers for grab-and-go options.

Invest in the Right Tools: Having the right kitchen tools can make meal prep much easier. Consider investing in:

- Food scale for portion control.

- Blender or food processor for making smoothies or sauces.
- Meal prep containers for storing pre-portioned meals.
- Spiralizer for creating veggie noodles as a low-carb alternative.

Batch Cooking: Dedicate one day a week to batch cooking. Prepare meals in advance and portion them out for the week. This saves time and ensures you have healthy options readily available.

Stay Hydrated: While not directly related to carb cycling, staying hydrated is crucial for overall health and can help curb cravings. Keep a water bottle handy and aim to drink at least 8 glasses of water a day.

Flexibility and Adjustment: Be flexible with your plan and listen to your body. If you find that a certain carb cycling approach isn't working for you, don't be afraid to adjust it. Everyone's body responds differently, so it may take some trial and error to find what works best for you.

By following these tips and setting up your kitchen for success, you'll be well-equipped to stick to your carb cycling plan and reach your health and fitness goals.

Understanding Your Body's Needs

Understanding your body's needs before starting carb cycling is crucial for optimizing your nutrition plan and achieving your fitness goals. Here's a breakdown of steps to help you better understand your body's requirements:

Assess Your Current Diet: Assessing your current diet involves keeping a detailed food journal for several days to gain insight into your eating habits. Record everything you consume, including portion sizes and timing, while also noting any physical or emotional responses after meals. This process fosters self-awareness, helping you identify patterns, triggers for unhealthy eating habits, and areas for improvement. By analyzing your current diet, you can pinpoint sources of nutrient deficiencies, excesses, or imbalances, guiding you toward more balanced and nutritious choices.

Additionally, assessing your diet allows you to recognize any tendencies toward emotional eating, mindless snacking, or reliance on processed foods. Armed with this information, you can make informed decisions about which dietary changes to prioritize and how to tailor your nutrition plan to better support your health and fitness goals. Whether aiming to lose weight, build muscle, or enhance overall well-being, understanding your starting point is essential for creating a realistic and effective strategy for long-term success.

Calculate Your Basal Metabolic Rate (BMR): Your Basal Metabolic Rate (BMR) is the foundational number of calories your body requires to sustain basic physiological functions while at rest. It represents the energy needed for vital processes such as breathing, circulation, and cell repair. Utilizing various formulas incorporating factors like age, gender, weight, height, and activity level, you can estimate your BMR accurately.

Numerous online calculators simplify this process, providing quick and accessible tools to gauge your BMR. Understanding your BMR serves as a cornerstone for developing personalized nutrition plans tailored to your energy needs. By aligning your calorie intake with your BMR, you establish a baseline for weight maintenance.

This knowledge also empowers you to make informed decisions about calorie deficits or surpluses necessary for weight loss or gain. Ultimately, comprehending your BMR aids in optimizing your dietary approach, ensuring that your nutritional intake aligns with your metabolic requirements for overall health and fitness goals.

Determine Your Total Daily Energy Expenditure (TDEE): Your TDEE accounts for your BMR plus the calories burned through physical activity and exercise. Knowing your TDEE helps you understand how many calories you need to maintain, gain, or lose weight.

Identify Your Goals: Are you looking to lose fat, gain muscle, improve athletic performance, or enhance overall health? Your goals will influence how you approach carb cycling and the balance of macronutrients (carbs, protein, and fats) in your diet.

Consider Your Activity Level: Your activity level plays a significant role in determining your carbohydrate needs. Those with higher activity levels or intense workout routines may require more carbs for energy replenishment and muscle recovery.

Assess Your Carb Tolerance: Pay attention to how your body responds to different levels of carbohydrate intake. Some individuals may thrive on higher carb days, while others feel better with lower carb intake. Experiment with different carb cycling patterns to find what works best for you.

Evaluate Your Relationship with Carbs: Consider your current relationship with carbohydrates. Are you sensitive to carb-induced energy crashes or cravings? Do you feel better with a steady supply of energy from complex carbs, or do you prefer a lower-carb, higher-fat approach? Understanding your preferences and tolerances can guide your carb cycling strategy.

Consult with a Professional: If you're unsure about how to assess your body's needs or create a carb cycling plan, consider consulting with a registered dietitian or nutritionist. They can provide personalized guidance based on your unique physiology, goals, and preferences.

By taking these steps to understand your body's needs before embarking on carb cycling, you can tailor your nutrition plan effectively, optimize your energy levels, and support your fitness journey.

Understanding the importance of protein intake or carbohydrate reduction is one thing, but without knowing your starting values or what defines an optimal ratio, managing your daily macros can prove challenging. This beginner-friendly guide aims to assist you in establishing a foundation for effectively managing your macros, creating a nutrition plan, and preparing meals that align with your macro requirements. While it doesn't cover every aspect of macros, this guide serves as a starting point to empower you in taking charge of your dietary choices.

Understanding your macros involves three key aspects:

1. Determining the appropriate macro ratio tailored to your requirements.
2. Planning your daily meals to achieve these macro ratios.
3. Implementing methods to accurately measure your macros.

While nutrition plays a crucial role in a healthy lifestyle, physical activity is equally essential for overall well-being.

Finding the Proper Ratio of Macros

Determining the optimal macro ratio involves identifying the percentage of your daily calorie intake allocated to protein, carbohydrates, and fats.

It's crucial to note that there's no universal set ratio. While one individual might thrive on a 40/40/20 ratio of proteins, carbs, and fats, another person may find a 40/50/10 ratio more suitable.

Moreover, your macro ratios are dynamic and should adapt to your goals. For instance, during a bulking phase, you might increase your carb intake, whereas during a cutting phase, reducing carbs may be beneficial.

Although there are starting guidelines like the aforementioned ratios, they serve as guides rather than rigid rules. Experiment with ratios such as 40/40/20 initially, and if you experience constant hunger, consider adjusting your macros.

If you notice a decrease in energy levels, increasing fats or carbs might be beneficial. Nutrition in bodybuilding blends science and art, aiming to strike the perfect balance between the two.

Planning Your Daily Diet – Breaking Down Your Macros

The first stage in designing your diet involves calculating your total daily energy expenditure (TDEE), which basically shows the number of calories the body needs. This value is affected by many of the factors such as age, gender, weight, metabolic rate, activity levels, goals and time in which the goals are set. There are loads of internet calculators, such as the one here, that can help you determine your TDEE. To make it easier, let's assume that your TDEP is 2,000 kcal/day and you are doing regular workouts without specific bulking or cutting programs.

Next you'll divide your macros to determine the adequate amount of calorie coming from each. On a 2000 calorie diet following the 40/40/20 plan, that means that you eat 800 calories from protein, 800 calories from carbs, and 400 calories from fats. Taking a calorie figure and dividing it by 4 will provide you with the exact amounts of macro needed in your daily diet.

To calculate your macros based on a 2,000-calorie diet, use the following conversions: you divide 800 calories for protein and carbs by 4 calories per gram to get 200 grams each. For fat divide 400 calories by 9 calories per gram to get around 44 g of fat (rounded down). For the case above, following the 40/40/20 ratio, try to consume 200g of protein, 200g of carbs, and 44g of fat daily.

How to Measure Your Macros?

As you delve into understanding macros and monitoring your food intake, it's essential to have three tools: a kitchen scale, a calorie/gram reference book or app, and measuring cups. Over time, you'll develop better skills in estimating portion sizes and recalling the protein, carbohydrate, or fat content of foods.

Utilizing these tools and recording your daily food intake will accelerate your progress by making you more accountable. This principle of accountability is evident in various domains, such as effective business management strategies and fitness regimens practiced by savvy bodybuilders striving for success in bodybuilding.

Now, where were we?

Although this calorie-counting book may seem comprehensive, we all in actual sense use a short list of 20-30 most favorite foods on a regular basis. Latterly, you will begin to remember such as a 6-ounce chicken breast containing approximately 140 calories, just over 26 grams of protein and 3 grams of fat. You will also be able to approximate the size of 6 ounces chicken breast without the need of weighing it on the kitchen scale.

For foods mostly measured by the ounce, like most meats, using a food scale is suggested. On the contrary, for foods measured by cups for calorie count, you will utilize your measuring cups. On the way, in a couple of weeks, you might be capable of preparing your weekly menus based on your notes. This brings us to the next step: planning your daily meals.

Planning your Meals with your Macros in Mind

Continuing with the above example of:

• 2,000 calorie diet for daily consumption.

• 40/40/20 breakdown

• 200g of protein, 200g of carbs and 44g of fat.

Imagine you are someone who works out in the morning, has to sit down for eight hours a day at work, and in the evening don't move much or sit at home. Unlike many people who are still struggling to lose or gain weight, they already achieved their goal which is maintaining their body. In the case with them, it is recommended to eat the bulk of their calories as well as carbs by 7 p. m. as they don't do evening exercises. In accordance to the individual-ness of dieting, rather than featuring certain foods, let's take into account a sample day's intake in grams. It is, however, necessary to acknowledge that this is a very broad outline.

A typical day's diet may look like this:

Breakfast:

- Scrambled eggs with veggies and a drizzle of olive oil, paired with a slice of whole-grain toast and a serving of fruit.

Protein: 30g

Carbohydrates: 60g

Fat: 10g

Post-Workout Protein Shake:

Protein: 20g

Carbohydrates: 30g

Fat: 2g

Morning Snack:

- Greek yogurt with mixed vegetables and a handful of nuts.

Protein: 20g

Carbohydrates: 20g

Fat: 10g

Lunch:

- Grilled chicken breast, steamed vegetables, and a portion of sweet potato.

Protein: 45g

Carbohydrates: 40g

Fat: 6g

Afternoon Snack:

- A piece of fruit paired with a slice of turkey or some low-fat dairy.

Protein: 25g

Carbohydrates: 20g

Fat: 2g

Dinner:

- Fish with a generous serving of roasted veggies and quinoa.

Protein: 45g

Carbohydrates: 30g

Fat: 8g

Evening Snack:

- A small piece of cold chicken and a side salad.

Protein: 15g

Fat: 4g

This breakdown provides a simplistic overview with approximate numbers for each meal, illustrating the concept.

Some Last Points to Remember

Don't get too caught up in precise calculations. Aim to get close to your macros, and when you're away from home or pressed for time, estimate your portions as accurately as possible. If your protein intake is slightly lower one day and your carb intake is a bit higher on another, don't stress about it. Avoid letting the pressure of achieving perfect macros dampen your motivation to eat healthily. Minor variations in ratios shouldn't be a cause for concern.

It's better to roughly follow a 40/40/20 ratio than to be unaware of what you're eating altogether. If you can't track everything every day, just do your best. Adjust your ratio if it leaves you feeling hungry or unable to complete your workouts. The key rule is to eat according to the ratio that suits your body best.

The Role of Proteins, Fats, and Carbohydrates

If you're dedicated to cycling, chances are you take nutrition seriously. You might meticulously track your daily calorie intake to ensure you're meeting the demands of your body.

So why, even if your total calorie consumption hasn't changed, do you suddenly feel like you lack enough energy for your long rides? Well, calories are more than just a simple number. Changing the source of those calories could significantly impact your cycling performance.

In essence, not all calories from protein, carbs, and fat are equal. To understand what this means for cyclists, we sought advice from our mentor, veteran cycling coach Darryl MacKenzie, who will guide you in choosing the right calories for optimal cycling performance.

The Complex Puzzle of Cycling Nutrition

Before delving into our cycling nutrition tips, it's essential to recognize one thing: Nutrition is intricate. Particularly for performance athletes like cyclists, there are numerous facets to consider. For instance, Lance Armstrong used to meticulously weigh every ingredient for his meals to ensure precise nutrition. It's impossible to cover every aspect in one go. What we're discussing here is just one facet of the broader picture. While crucial for your cycling achievements, there's much more depth to explore. Keep this in mind and consider consulting a nutritionist for comprehensive guidance on crafting a carb cycling workout plan.

Not All Calories Are Created Equal

Here's your initial step in selecting the appropriate calories for cycling. In nutrition, a cyclist must go beyond the fundamental balance of calories in versus calories out. While this principle aids in weight maintenance, it's inadequate for optimizing cycling performance.

"For cyclists, the value derived from protein isn't the same as that from carbs," Coach Darryl clarifies. "And the value from fat differs from that of carbs."

However, the differentiation extends further. Protein, carbs, and fat serve distinct purposes for your body:

- Protein aids in muscle rebuilding and restoration.
- Carbs supply readily usable energy.
- Fats contribute to your body's fat stores, providing insulation and energy reserves for when needed.

Plan the Right Calories for the Right Time

"The timing of your food intake matters," emphasizes Darryl. To align your nutrition with your cycling objectives, especially for long-distance cycling, strategic timing of different calorie types is crucial.

While fats can be a regular part of your diet in appropriate quantities, they don't offer specific benefits for cyclists. However, it's important to note that every gram of fat provides over twice the calories of protein or carbohydrates. Thus, if weight loss is your cycling goal, monitoring fat intake is essential. However, the timing is paramount for carbs and protein. The rule is straightforward: consume carbs before riding and protein afterward.

Eating a heavy steak the day before a ride isn't beneficial. It diverts your body's energy towards digesting the meat rather than efficiently fueling your ride. Instead, for a weekend of cycling, load up on carbs on Friday night and Saturday morning, ensuring quick carb intake during the ride with sports drinks. Save protein consumption for Sunday night and Monday to aid muscle recovery.

Looking ahead to your next ride, remember that not all calories are equal. Focus on fine-tuning your diet composition and timing, not just total calorie intake. Coach Darryl assures that these adjustments will make a noticeable difference in your cycling performance.

What are macronutrients?

Food nutrients are divided into two main categories based on the body's requirement levels: macronutrients and micronutrients. Macronutrients are essential in larger quantities and include carbohydrates, fat, and protein. On the other hand, micronutrients, such as vitamins and minerals, are needed in smaller amounts.

Macronutrients play a crucial role in providing energy to the body. Additionally, they contribute to insulation against cold temperatures, ensure proper cellular function, and support the activity of gut microbes.

What are carbohydrates?

Therefore, carbohydrates are fundamental in your diet as they are the primary source of body energy that you cannot do without. They offer glucose to your cells by acting as a source of fuel. Similarly, complex carbohydrates like fiber sustain the proper functionality of your gut microbiota. Carbohydrates can be found in many foods.

Their effect on health is however not uniform but rather depends on the source. The main dietary carbohydrates are of three types. They all play their different roles in the body.

Sugars: The complex macromolecules glucose, fructose, and sucrose are called sugar. These particles are taken up by the cells all over your body, and then they can be used to provide energy to these cells.

Starches: In contrast, more complex carbohydrate molecules – most notably starches – are digested over a longer period of time than sugars. Your system must now complex carbohydrates into simple sugars so that cells can use these for energy supply. These periods of low intensity lead to a more consistent flow of energy being delivered into the bloodstream.

Fiber: Fiber is not digested by human enzymes and is classified as a form of carbohydrate molecule, but it cannot be fully digested by the body. Different fiber molecules of diets help your health a lot. Microbiota of the abdomen make fiber into short-chain fatty acids (SCFAs) which are important for maintaining blood sugar level, blood fat level and appetite. For instance, SCFAs likewise play a role in the health of your immune system by helping sustain your gut microbiome.

Best sources of carbohydrates

Scientific research highlights that the healthiest carbohydrate sources are found in unprocessed or minimally processed foods. These foods typically combine sugars, starches, and fiber along with essential vitamins, minerals, and plant antioxidants known as phytonutrients, which combat inflammation. The degree of food processing significantly impacts its health benefits. In contrast, ultra processed foods often contain high levels of refined carbohydrates, added sugars, salt, unhealthy fats, or artificial additives that lack essential nutrients for the body.

For instance, consider the contrast between carbohydrates in a slice of apple pie and a whole apple. The pie contains processed carbohydrates like sugar and butter, which are not naturally present. This raises the question: why is eating the whole apple healthier? It's due to its higher fiber and starch content compared to sugar. Notably, whole fruits and milk provide a range of nutrients, while table sugar solely serves as an energy source.

Regarding carbohydrate sources, key options include whole grains, fruits, vegetables, legumes, and nuts and seeds. Opting for high-quality carbohydrates is crucial not only to nourish your body but also to support the health of your gut microbiota, thereby promoting overall well-being.

What is fat?

Fat, a vital nutrient for overall health, is composed of fat molecules or triglycerides containing glycerol, a sugar alcohol, and three fatty acids. Like carbohydrates, fat acts as an energy source, helps in insulation to regulate body temperature, aids in the absorption of fat-soluble vitamins A, D, E, and K, and supplies essential fatty acids like omega-3. Omega-3, important for brain health, cannot be synthesized by the body, underscoring the necessity of fat for the proper functioning of every cell in your body.

There are three main types of dietary fat:

Monounsaturated and polyunsaturated fats are both counted as unsaturated fats that remain liquid when being placed at a room temperature and known to provide health benefits for the body. These include cases in which omega-3, a polyunsaturated fat with diverse health benefits including heart health support and the reduced mortality risk as proven by current research.

The fat molecules in animal products and some plants are in solid form at room temperature (saturated fats). Originally, these types of diets were associated with a higher risk profile of heart diseases, inflammation, and bad cholesterol levels. Nevertheless, the association between saturated fats and heart health has been questioned in recent studies, thus demonstrating a more complex relationship between these two aspects.

Artificial fats, also known as partially hydrogenated oils, are synthetically produced by the process of transforming vegetable oils. Although beef and dairy fat have small amounts of natural trans fat, consuming trans fats, mainly in the artificial kind, results in a raft of health problems including elevated cholesterol, increased inflammation, and insulin resistance. Although partially hydrogenated oils are prohibited to produce ultra-processed and fast foods in the U. S. , these oils are still in the production of numerous ultra-processed and fast foods in the U. K.

Best sources of fat

The quality of fat you consume is crucial for your body's optimal functioning. Processed fats can alter your body's response to food. Opting for unsaturated fats is the healthiest choice. Although recent research is shifting perspectives on saturated fats, adhering to moderate consumption aligns with official dietary recommendations. Low-fat dairy products frequently include added sugar, potentially leading to weight gain and disrupting blood sugar regulation. Choosing full-fat dairy, despite its saturated fat content, can sometimes be a healthier option than low-fat alternatives.

What is protein?

Proteins consist of long chains of amino acids and play crucial roles in maintaining health. They serve various functions within your body, including acting as enzymes that catalyze chemical reactions, producing neurotransmitters, hormones, and antibodies. While proteins can be a source of energy, their primary role lies in cellular repair and growth, especially post-exercise. Including adequate protein in your diet is essential for overall balance.

The body utilizes more than 20 amino acids; through unique combinations of two or more of them, these amino acids form hundreds of proteins in the organism. On this list of the amino acids, there are nine essential ones. This means that your body is not able to manufacture them, therefore you must receive them in your body through food sources.

There are two different types of protein sources:

Complete Proteins: Complete proteins are characterized by the fact they contain all nine essential amino acids, being mainly of animal origin, like beef, chicken, and fish. Some vegetable substitutions are equally complete proteins, like quinoa and soy.

Incomplete Proteins: As a rule of thumb, incomplete proteins lack one or more of the essential amino acids and most heavily appear in plant-based protein sources, such as beans, pulses, seeds, nuts, and whole grains. Taking in a sufficient number of these foods is critical to acquire much-needed amino acids.

Best sources of protein

When it comes to proteins, opting for minimally processed, high-quality sources is ideal for your health.

Here are some high-quality protein sources to consider:

- Tofu
- Beans

- Eggs
- Nuts and seeds
- Legumes
- Dairy
- Fish
- Tempeh

Diet quality is key

Feeling guilty after enjoying your favorite treat is a common experience, but it's important not to stress over occasional indulgences. Instead of fixating on every food item, prioritize the overall quality of your diet. Quality dieting goes beyond trendy eating plans, offering a holistic view of your nutritional intake rather than micromanaging each meal component.

Macronutrients, including carbohydrates, fats, and proteins, are vital nutrients your body requires in significant quantities for energy and various bodily functions. Rather than focusing solely on tracking macronutrient levels, concentrate on maintaining a nutritious overall diet. Everyone responds uniquely to different foods, so understanding your individual dietary needs enables you to eat for optimal health instead of adhering strictly to generic dietary guidelines.

Calculating Your Daily Needs

Understanding your body's daily calorie requirements is pivotal for effective weight management, whether your goal is shedding pounds, packing on muscle, or maintaining your current weight. These needs encompass vital bodily functions such as respiration, digestion, and circulation—essentially the energy baseline required for sustaining life. Employing the Harris-Benedict formula serves as a compass for adjusting your calorie intake, ensuring it aligns with your weight management objectives.

The Harris-Benedict formula unveils your Basal Metabolic Rate (BMR), essentially the foundational energy expenditure for your body at rest. This figure is influenced not only by factors like gender, age, and body composition but also by the stationary state of the body, representing the calories burned daily. The computation of BMR involves a series of steps.

Step 1: Determining Your BMR

- For Women: BMR = 655 + (9.563 × weight in kg) + (1.850 × height in cm) - (4.676 × age in years)
- For Men: BMR = 66.47 + (13.75 × weight in kg) + (5.003 × height in cm) - (6.755 × age in years)

Your Active Metabolic Rate (AMR) kicks in when you factor in your activity level, adjusting your baseline metabolic rate to reflect your daily physical exertion. This adjustment involves multiplying your BMR by a specific factor based on your activity level, ranging from 1.2 (sedentary) to 1.9 (very active), to arrive at your AMR.

Step 2: Determining Your AMR

The AMR adjustments based on activity levels are as follows:

- Sedentary (little or no exercise): AMR = BMR × 1.2
- Lightly active (exercise 1–3 days/week): AMR = BMR × 1.375
- Moderately active (exercise 3–5 days/week): AMR = BMR × 1.55
- Active (exercise 6–7 days/week): AMR = BMR × 1.725
- Very active (hard exercise 6–7 days/week): AMR = BMR × 1.9

Your daily caloric intake represents the energy required to maintain your current weight. Weight loss or gain can be achieved by either adjusting your physical activity levels or modifying your daily calorie intake.

For effective weight loss planning, understanding your AMR is crucial, as it delineates the calorie deficit needed to reach your target weight. For instance, if your BMR is 1,400 (the average for American women) and you're moderately active, your AMR would be 2,170 (1,400 × 1.55). Considering that burning 7,000 calories equates to shedding a pound of fat per week, a daily deficit of 500 calories is recommended.

In a non-exercise weight loss scenario, your daily calorie intake would need to be 1,670 (2,170 - 500 = 1,670). Alternatively, you could achieve the same deficit by burning an additional 500 calories through exercise. The adage "you are what you eat" rings true; combining a balanced diet with regular exercise typically yields the most effective results in weight management endeavors.

Adjusting Your Intake: When and How

Adjusting your intake is a nuanced art, requiring careful consideration of when and how you consume calories to align with your health and fitness goals. Whether your aim is to shed excess weight, build muscle, or simply maintain a balanced lifestyle, strategic adjustments to your dietary habits can make a significant difference.

Timing plays a crucial role in optimizing your calorie consumption. Starting your day with a nutritious breakfast kick-starts your metabolism and provides the energy needed to fuel your activities. Aim for a balanced meal that includes protein, healthy fats, and complex carbohydrates to sustain you through the morning.

Throughout the day, spacing out your meals and snacks can help maintain stable blood sugar levels and prevent energy crashes. Consider incorporating smaller, frequent meals to keep hunger at bay and avoid overeating during main meals. Listen to your body's hunger cues and eat when you're genuinely hungry, rather than out of habit or boredom.

In the evening, be mindful of portion sizes and avoid heavy, calorie-laden meals close to bedtime, as this can interfere with digestion and disrupt sleep. Opt for lighter, nutrient-dense options to support restful sleep and proper overnight recovery.

How to Adjust Your Intake?

When it comes to adjusting your calorie intake, moderation and balance are key. Rather than resorting to drastic measures or restrictive diets, focus on making sustainable changes that you can maintain in the long term.

One approach is to practice mindful eating, paying attention to your body's hunger and fullness signals and eating in response to physical hunger rather than emotional triggers. This can help prevent overeating and promote a healthier relationship with food.

Another strategy is to prioritize nutrient-dense foods that provide essential vitamins, minerals, and antioxidants while limiting empty calories from processed foods and sugary snacks. Incorporating plenty of fruits, vegetables, lean proteins, whole grains, and healthy fats into your diet can help satisfy hunger and support overall health and well-being.

Additionally, consider keeping a food journal to track your intake and identify patterns or areas where adjustments may be needed. This can help increase awareness of your eating habits and empower you to make more informed choices.

Ultimately, adjusting your intake is a personal journey that requires experimentation and self-discovery. By listening to your body, practicing moderation, and making gradual changes over time, you can find a dietary approach that supports your health and fitness goals while enjoying a satisfying and fulfilling relationship with food.

Must Read!!!

Thank you for choosing to explore my book! Your support means the world to me. As a valued reader, your review holds immense significance. Your insights not only guide potential readers but also contribute to shaping the ongoing journey of this book. Your thoughts help in fostering a community of engaged readers, making the experience richer for everyone.

How You Can Share Your Review?

Sharing your review on Amazon allows others to benefit from your perspective, aiding them in their decision-making process.

To post your review, simply visit the Amazon page where you discovered my book, head to the 'Customer Reviews' section, and click on 'Write a customer review' to share your invaluable feedback.

Alternatively, you can effortlessly access the review section by scanning the QR code below with your smartphone. Thank you once again for your support and for considering sharing your thoughts with us.

Chapter 4: The Carb Cycling Blueprint

Carb cycling might sound simple in theory: keeping in mind having high-carb and low-carb days under your belt or not matter so much because the body's glycogen is concerned, not the way it uses carbs. For example, one can get carried away by running 5km every day without following a clear plan to manage this cycle could become very stressful. With consumption of carb-cycling dieting plan, you will not only get rid of confusion but also find yourself on a clear road for your dietary direction.

Meal plan if it is for all and not only the people who wish to accomplish a certain purpose in nutrition. It has doesn't need be complicated or time-consuming. Simple measures you might borrow include skipping meals for the sake of proper meal structures, making shopping lists and food. Amongst these you can reduce food waste, save more and meet your nutrition needs.

Carb cycling refers to the way of tuning-up your carb intake into the workout and away from the workout. On lowactivity days, carbohydrate uptake is also decreased that is rest days. Similarly, on the days when you are active, for example, you are working out or need more calories than usual, you will be adding additional carbs as well. It makes the training planning flexible and user-friendly based on your training scheme and needs. Different from constant low-carb dieting that results in suboptimal performance and energy states, carb cycling helps to optimize energy level and prevent drop of performance stage through exercise.

To make sure you're having enough carbs on high-carb days, consider adding up to about 50% of your carbohydrate intake to your total calorie intake. On low-carb days please do not reduce the calories from carbs percentage to less than 10% to 15% of the total calorie intake. Many opinions exist about what kind of diet plan will work better: higher protein lower carb, or vice versa; higher fat lower.

Overview of the 4-Week Plan

Carb cycling is a dietary approach that involves alternating between high-carb and low-carb days to optimize performance, promote fat loss, and maintain muscle mass. This 4-week plan provides a structured framework for implementing carb cycling effectively.

Week 1:

- Start with three low-carb days followed by one high-carb day.
- Focus on lean protein sources, vegetables, and healthy fats on low-carb days.
- On high-carb days, incorporate complex carbohydrates such as whole grains, fruits, and starchy vegetables to replenish glycogen stores and support intense workouts.

Week 2:

- Adjust the ratio to two low-carb days followed by two high-carb days.
- Continue to prioritize nutrient-dense foods on both low and high-carb days, while adjusting portion sizes to align with energy needs and fitness goals.

Week 3:

- Maintain a balanced approach with alternating low and high-carb days.
- Experiment with timing and distribution of carbohydrates around workouts to optimize energy levels and recovery.

Week 4:

- Fine-tune carb cycling based on individual preferences and responses.
- Monitor progress, adjust macronutrient ratios as needed, and focus on sustainability for long-term success.

Throughout the 4-week plan, it's essential to stay hydrated, prioritize quality sleep, and listen to your body's hunger and satiety cues. Consistency, flexibility, and mindful eating are key principles of the carb cycling blueprint, helping you achieve your health and fitness goals while enjoying a balanced and sustainable approach to nutrition.

High Carb Days Explained

High carb days are an integral part of carb cycling, strategically incorporated to replenish glycogen stores, boost energy levels, and support muscle growth and recovery. During high carb days, individuals consume a higher proportion of carbohydrates compared to low carb days, typically accounting for a significant portion of their total daily calorie intake.

The Science of High Carb Days:

High carb days are a fundamental component of carb cycling, a dietary strategy that involves alternating between periods of higher and lower carbohydrate intake. Understanding the science behind high carb days involves delving into how carbohydrates are utilized by the body for energy, glycogen replenishment, and metabolic regulation.

Glycogen Replenishment: Carbohydrates are the body's primary source of energy, particularly during intense physical activity. When you consume carbohydrates, they are broken down into glucose, which is either used immediately for energy or stored in the liver and muscles as glycogen for later use. During periods of low carb intake or intense exercise, glycogen stores become depleted. High carb days provide an opportunity to replenish these glycogen stores, ensuring that the body has an adequate fuel source for future workouts and activities.

Insulin Regulation: Carbohydrates stimulate the release of insulin, a hormone produced by the pancreas that helps regulate blood sugar levels. When you consume carbohydrates, blood glucose levels rise, prompting the pancreas to release insulin to facilitate the uptake of glucose into cells. Insulin also plays a crucial role in promoting glycogen synthesis, muscle protein synthesis, and inhibiting the breakdown of muscle tissue. High carb days, which involve a higher intake of carbohydrates, result in increased insulin secretion, promoting glycogen storage and anabolism (muscle building).

Hormonal Balance: High carb days can influence various hormones involved in metabolism, appetite regulation, and energy expenditure. For example, leptin, known as the "satiety hormone," is produced by fat cells and helps signal fullness to the brain, potentially reducing appetite and preventing overeating. Ghrelin, on the other hand, is known as the "hunger hormone" and stimulates appetite. High carb days may help regulate these hormones, leading to improved appetite control and reduced cravings.

Muscle Growth and Recovery: Carbohydrates play a critical role in supporting muscle growth, repair, and recovery, especially after strenuous exercise. Consuming carbohydrates post-workout helps replenish glycogen stores and provides the necessary energy for muscle repair and protein synthesis. By strategically incorporating high carb days into a carb cycling regimen, individuals can optimize muscle recovery and adaptation to training stimuli.

Overall, the science of high carb days revolves around optimizing carbohydrate intake to support energy needs, glycogen replenishment, hormonal balance, and muscle growth and recovery. By understanding these physiological processes, individuals can tailor their nutrition strategies to align with their goals, whether it's improving athletic performance, supporting muscle growth, or promoting overall health and well-being.

Best Practices for High Carb Meals:

To maximize the benefits of high carb days, it's essential to focus on consuming complex carbohydrates from nutrient-dense sources rather than simple sugars or processed foods. Opt for whole grains, legumes, fruits, and starchy vegetables, which provide a steady release of energy and a wealth of vitamins, minerals, and fiber.

Timing is also crucial on high carb days, with many individuals preferring to consume the majority of their carbohydrates around workouts to fuel performance and promote recovery. This approach ensures that the body efficiently utilizes carbohydrates for energy rather than storing them as fat.

Balancing high carb meals with adequate protein and healthy fats can further enhance satiety, stabilize blood sugar levels, and support muscle repair and growth. Incorporating lean protein sources such as chicken, fish, tofu, or legumes alongside carbohydrates can help optimize the nutrient composition of meals on high carb days.

Lastly, mindful portion control and listening to hunger cues are essential on high carb days to prevent overeating and maintain a healthy balance of macronutrients. Pay attention to how different carbohydrate sources affect your energy levels and performance, and adjust your intake accordingly to suit your individual needs and preferences.

Low Carb Days Unpacked

Low carb days are pivotal components of carb cycling, a dietary regimen involving alternating between periods of higher and lower carbohydrate intake. During these days, individuals purposefully reduce their carbohydrate consumption, with a focus on deriving calories primarily from protein and fat sources. By limiting carbs, the body is prompted to utilize alternative fuel sources, such as stored fat, leading to a state of ketosis where fat breakdown is increased for energy production.

This metabolic shift not only promotes fat loss but also stabilizes blood sugar levels, curbing cravings and aiding in adherence to a calorie-controlled diet. Low carb days also improve insulin sensitivity, facilitating the mobilization and utilization of stored fat for energy. To succeed on low carb days, planning meals in advance, emphasizing protein and healthy fats, including non-starchy vegetables, staying hydrated, monitoring portion sizes, and listening to hunger cues are key strategies. By consistently following these practices, individuals can optimize fat loss and progress towards their health and fitness objectives effectively.

Tips for Succeeding on Low Carb Days

Plan Meals in Advance: Prepare meals and snacks ahead of time to ensure you have low carb options readily available. This can help prevent impulsive food choices and keep you on track with your dietary goals.

Focus on Protein and Healthy Fats: Prioritize protein-rich foods such as lean meats, poultry, fish, eggs, and plant-based sources like tofu and legumes. Incorporate healthy fats from sources such as avocados, nuts, seeds, olive oil, and fatty fish to promote satiety and support overall health.

Include Non-Starchy Vegetables: Non-starchy vegetables like leafy greens, broccoli, cauliflower, and bell peppers are low in carbohydrates but high in fiber, vitamins, and minerals. They can add volume and nutrient density to meals without significantly increasing carbohydrate intake.

Stay Hydrated: Drink plenty of water throughout the day to stay hydrated and support metabolic processes. Aim to consume at least eight glasses of water daily, and consider incorporating herbal teas or flavored water for variety.

Monitor Portion Sizes: Pay attention to portion sizes, particularly when consuming higher calorie foods like nuts, cheese, and oils. While these foods are nutritious, they are also calorie-dense, so it's essential to practice portion control to avoid overeating.

Listen to Your Body: Pay attention to hunger and satiety cues, and adjust your food intake accordingly. Experiment with meal timing and frequency to find a pattern that works best for your body and lifestyle.

By implementing these strategies and staying consistent with your low carb approach, you can maximize fat loss potential and progress toward your health and fitness goals effectively.

Cheat Days: Myths and Facts

Cheat days have become a common topic in discussions about dieting and weight loss, but there are several misconceptions surrounding them. Let's unravel the myths and present the facts about cheat days:

Myth: Cheat days are necessary for weight loss success. Fact: While some people find that occasional indulgences help them stick to their overall diet plan, cheat days aren't essential for everyone. Consistently following a balanced, nutritious diet and maintaining a healthy lifestyle is key to long-term weight loss success.

Myth: Cheat days can undo all your progress. Fact: Enjoying a treat or indulging in a favorite food occasionally is unlikely to derail your progress if it's done in moderation. What matters most is your overall dietary pattern and lifestyle habits. If you find that cheat days lead to overindulgence or feelings of guilt, it may be helpful to reframe them as planned indulgences or special occasions.

Myth: Cheat days promote an unhealthy relationship with food. Fact: For some individuals, rigid dietary rules can lead to feelings of deprivation and guilt around food. Allowing yourself occasional treats can actually help foster a more balanced approach to eating and reduce the likelihood of binge eating or emotional eating episodes. It's important to practice moderation and mindfulness when incorporating treats into your diet.

Myth: Cheat days are an excuse to overeat unhealthy foods. Fact: While cheat days often involve indulging in foods that are higher in calories or less nutritious, they don't have to be synonymous with unhealthy eating. You can still enjoy treats in moderation while prioritizing nutrient-dense foods the majority of the time. Opting for healthier versions of your favorite treats or practicing portion control can help you enjoy your indulgences without feeling deprived.

Myth: Cheat days can boost metabolism. Fact: There's limited scientific evidence to support the idea that occasional splurges can significantly impact metabolism. While a temporary increase in calorie intake may slightly elevate metabolic rate due to the thermic effect of food, any effects are likely to be short-lived and negligible in the context of overall weight loss efforts.

In summary, while cheat days can be a part of some people's dietary approach, they're not a one-size-fits-all solution for weight loss or maintenance. It's essential to approach them mindfully, focusing on balance, moderation, and enjoyment without letting them undermine your overall health and wellness goals.

Breakfast Recipes

Banana Oat Pancakes Recipe

Ingredients:

- 1 cup of rolled oats

- 2 ripe bananas (mashed)

- 2 eggs

- 1 teaspoon of baking powder

- ½ teaspoon of cinnamon

Instructions:

1. Combine rolled oats, mashed bananas, eggs, baking powder, and cinnamon in a blender and blend until smooth.

2. Preheat a non-stick skillet over medium heat and lightly grease it with cooking spray or oil.

3. Pour the pancake batter onto the skillet to create pancakes of your desired size.

4. Cook the pancakes until bubbles form on the surface, then flip them and cook until both sides are golden brown.

Time Details:

- Prep Time: 5 minutes

- Cook Time: 10 minutes

- Total Time: 15 minutes

Blueberry Muffins with Honey Recipe

Ingredients:

- 1 ½ cups of all-purpose flour

- ½ cup of blueberries

- ¼ cup of honey

- ¼ cup of milk

- ¼ cup of melted butter

- 1 egg

- 1 teaspoon of baking powder

- ½ teaspoon of salt

Instructions:

1. Begin by preheating your oven to 375°F (190°C) and preparing a muffin tin with paper liners.
2. In a mixing bowl, whisk together flour, baking powder, and salt until well combined.
3. In another bowl, blend honey, milk, melted butter, and egg until smooth.
4. Combine the wet ingredients with the dry ingredients, stirring until just mixed. Gently fold in the blueberries.
5. Evenly distribute the batter among the muffin cups in the prepared tin.
6. Bake for 18-20 minutes or until a toothpick inserted into the center of a muffin comes out clean.

Time Details:

- Prep Time: 10 minutes

- Cook Time: 18-20 minutes

- Total Time: 28-30 minutes

Maple and Brown Sugar Oatmeal

Ingredients:

- 1 cup rolled oats
- 2 cups water
- 2 tablespoons maple syrup
- 2 tablespoons brown sugar

Instructions:

1. In a saucepan, bring water to a boil.
2. Stir in rolled oats and reduce heat to medium-low. Cook for 5 minutes, stirring occasionally.
3. Stir in maple syrup and brown sugar until well combined.

4. Remove from heat and let it sit for a minute before serving.

Prep Time: 1 minute

Cook Time: 5 minutes

Total Time: 6 minutes

Sweet Potato and Black Bean Breakfast Burritos

Ingredients:

- 2 large sweet potatoes, diced
- 1 can black beans, drained and rinsed
- 6 large eggs, scrambled
- 6 large flour tortillas
- Salt and pepper to taste
- Optional toppings: salsa, avocado, shredded cheese, sour cream

Instructions:

1. Begin by heating a skillet over medium heat and adding diced sweet potatoes. Cook them until they are tender, which should take about 10-12 minutes.

2. Next, add black beans to the skillet and cook them along with the sweet potatoes for an additional 2-3 minutes.

3. Warm up the tortillas either in the microwave or on a skillet.

4. Once the tortillas are warm, divide the sweet potato and black bean mixture among them. Top each with scrambled eggs and any other desired toppings.

5. Roll up the tortillas, making sure to tuck in the sides as you go, to create delicious burritos.

Prep Time: 10 minutes

Cook Time: 15 minutes

Total Time: 25 minutes

Customization: You can customize these burritos by adding ingredients like diced bell peppers, onions, spinach, or your favorite hot sauce for extra flavor.

Apple Cinnamon French toast

Ingredients:

- 6 slices of bread
- 3 eggs
- 1/2 cup milk
- 1 teaspoon vanilla extract
- 1 teaspoon ground cinnamon
- 1 apple, thinly sliced
- Butter or oil for frying
- Maple syrup for serving

Instructions:

1. Start by whisking together eggs, milk, vanilla extract, and cinnamon in a shallow bowl.

2. Dip each slice of bread into the egg mixture, ensuring both sides are evenly coated.

3. Heat butter or oil in a skillet over medium heat and place the dipped bread slices in the skillet.

4. Cook the bread until it turns golden brown on both sides, approximately 2-3 minutes per side.

5. Serve the French toast topped with sliced apples and drizzled with maple syrup for a delicious breakfast treat.

Prep Time: 5 minutes

Cook Time: 10 minutes

Total Time: 15 minutes

Customization: Add a sprinkle of powdered sugar or a dollop of whipped cream for extra sweetness.

Quinoa and Fruit Breakfast Bowl

Ingredients:

- 1 cup cooked quinoa
- Assorted fruits (such as berries, sliced bananas, diced mango)
- Honey or maple syrup for drizzling
- Greek yogurt or milk for serving

Instructions:

1. Divide cooked quinoa into bowls.
2. Top with assorted fruits of your choice.
3. Drizzle with honey or maple syrup.
4. Serve with a dollop of Greek yogurt or milk on the side.

Prep Time: 5 minutes

Total Time: 5 minutes

Customization: Feel free to mix and match fruits based on what's in season or your personal preferences. You can also add nuts or seeds for extra crunch.

Cranberry Almond Granola

Ingredients:

- 3 cups rolled oats
- 1 cup sliced almonds
- 1/2 cup dried cranberries
- 1/4 cup honey
- 1/4 cup coconut oil, melted
- 1 teaspoon vanilla extract

Instructions:

1. Begin by preheating your oven to 300°F (150°C) and lining a baking sheet with parchment paper.

2. In a large bowl, combine rolled oats, sliced almonds, and dried cranberries.

3. In another bowl, whisk together honey, melted coconut oil, and vanilla extract.

4. Pour the wet ingredients over the dry ingredients in the large bowl, stirring until everything is evenly coated.

5. Spread the mixture evenly onto the prepared baking sheet.

6. Bake for 25-30 minutes, remembering to stir halfway through, until the granola turns golden brown and becomes crisp.

7. Once baked, allow the granola to cool completely before transferring it to an airtight container for storage.

Prep Time: 5 minutes

Cook Time: 25-30 minutes

Total Time: 30-35 minutes

Customization: Customize your granola by adding other dried fruits, such as raisins or apricots, or swapping almonds for your favorite nuts like pecans or walnuts.

Pumpkin Spice Waffles

Ingredients:

- 2 cups all-purpose flour
- 1/4 cup packed brown sugar
- 1 tablespoon baking powder
- 1 teaspoon ground cinnamon
- 1/2 teaspoon ground nutmeg
- 1/4 teaspoon ground cloves
- 1/4 teaspoon salt
- 1 3/4 cups milk
- 1/2 cup pumpkin puree
- 1/4 cup unsalted butter, melted
- 2 large eggs
- 1 teaspoon vanilla extract

Instructions:

1. Begin by preheating your waffle iron following the instructions provided by the manufacturer.

2. In a large bowl, whisk together flour, brown sugar, baking powder, cinnamon, nutmeg, cloves, and salt until well combined.

3. In another bowl, combine milk, pumpkin puree, melted butter, eggs, and vanilla extract, whisking until the mixture is thoroughly blended.

4. Pour the wet ingredients into the bowl with the dry ingredients, stirring until just combined. Be careful not to overmix.

5. Using a ladle, pour the batter into the preheated waffle iron and cook according to the manufacturer's instructions until the waffles are golden and crisp.

Prep Time: 10 minutes

Cook Time: 10 minutes

Total Time: 20 minutes

Customization: You can add chopped nuts or chocolate chips to the batter for extra texture and flavor. Serve with whipped cream and a drizzle of maple syrup for a delightful treat.

Caramelized Pear and Brie Crepes

Ingredients:

- 1 cup all-purpose flour
- 2 eggs
- 1/2 cup milk
- 1/2 cup water
- 2 tablespoons unsalted butter, melted
- Pinch of salt
- 2 ripe pears, thinly sliced
- 4 ounces Brie cheese, sliced
- 1/4 cup caramel sauce

Instructions:

1. Place flour, eggs, milk, water, melted butter, and salt in a blender and blend until a smooth batter forms.

2. Heat a non-stick skillet over medium heat and lightly grease it with butter or oil.

3. Pour a small amount of the batter into the skillet, swirling it around to coat the bottom evenly. Cook for approximately 1-2 minutes until the edges start to lift.

4. Carefully flip the crepe and cook the other side for another 1-2 minutes until it turns golden brown. Repeat this process with the remaining batter.

5. Fill each crepe with sliced pears and Brie cheese, folding or rolling them up.

6. Just before serving, drizzle caramel sauce generously over the crepes for added flavor.

Prep Time: 15 minutes

Cook Time: 20 minutes

Total Time: 35 minutes

Customization: You can substitute pears with other fruits like apples or berries. Feel free to use different types of cheese, such as goat cheese or cream cheese, for variation.

Bagel with Cream Cheese and Smoked Salmon

Ingredients:

- 2 bagels, sliced and toasted
- 4 ounces cream cheese
- 4 ounces smoked salmon
- Thinly sliced red onion
- Capers (optional)
- Fresh dill (optional)

Instructions:

1. Spread cream cheese generously on each toasted bagel half.

2. Top with smoked salmon slices, red onion slices, capers, and fresh dill, if desired.

3. Serve immediately and enjoy!

Prep Time: 5 minutes

Total Time: 5 minutes

Customization: You can customize your bagel by adding ingredients like sliced tomatoes, cucumber, or avocado. Experiment with different types of cream cheese flavors, such as herb or garlic, for added taste.

Cherry and Almond Porridge

Ingredients:

- 1 cup rolled oats
- 2 cups milk (or water for a lighter option)
- 1/2 cup fresh or frozen cherries, pitted and halved
- 1/4 cup sliced almonds
- 2 tablespoons honey or maple syrup
- Pinch of salt

Instructions:

1. Start by bringing milk or water to a gentle simmer in a saucepan over medium heat.

2. Add rolled oats to the simmering liquid, then reduce the heat to low. Cook the oats for approximately 5-7 minutes, stirring occasionally, until they become tender and the mixture thickens.

3. Incorporate fresh or frozen cherries into the oatmeal and continue cooking for an additional 2-3 minutes until the cherries are heated through.

4. Take the saucepan off the heat and add sliced almonds, along with a drizzle of honey or maple syrup, and a pinch of salt for flavor enhancement.

5. Divide the prepared porridge among serving bowls and serve it hot.

Prep Time: 5 minutes

Cook Time: 10 minutes

Total Time: 15 minutes

Customization: You can customize your porridge by using different types of fruit such as berries, sliced bananas, or diced apples. Add a sprinkle of cinnamon or nutmeg for extra flavor.

Raspberry Yogurt Parfait

Ingredients:

- 1 cup Greek yogurt
- 1/2 cup fresh raspberries
- 1/4 cup granola
- 1 tablespoon honey

Instructions:

1. In a serving glass or bowl, layer Greek yogurt, fresh raspberries, and granola.
2. Drizzle honey over the top.
3. Repeat the layers until the glass or bowl is filled.
4. Serve immediately as a delicious and nutritious breakfast or snack.

Prep Time: 5 minutes

Total Time: 5 minutes

Personalization: Tailor your parfait to your preferences by opting for various yogurt options like vanilla or flavored varieties. Swap out raspberries for alternative fruits like strawberries, blueberries, or sliced peaches. Explore different granola types or incorporate nuts and seeds for added texture and flavor.

Lunch Recipes
Quinoa Salad with Roasted Sweet Potatoes and Apples

Ingredients:

- Quinoa
- Sweet potatoes
- Apples
- Mixed greens
- Olive oil
- Balsamic vinegar
- Salt and pepper

Instructions:

1. Prepare quinoa following the instructions on the package.

2. Cut sweet potatoes and apples into cubes, coat them with olive oil, salt, and pepper, and roast until they are tender.

3. Combine the cooked quinoa, roasted sweet potatoes and apples, and mixed greens to create the salad.

4. Drizzle balsamic vinegar over the salad, toss it gently, and then serve.

Prep Time: 15 minutes

Cook Time: 25 minutes

Total Time: 40 minutes

Customization: Add nuts (like pecans or walnuts) or dried cranberries for extra flavor and texture.

Vegetarian Sushi Rolls

Ingredients:

- Sushi rice
- Nori sheets
- Avocado
- Cucumber
- Carrots
- Bell peppers
- Sesame seeds
- Soy sauce (for dipping)

Instructions:

0. Prepare sushi rice following the instructions on the package and allow it to cool.

1. Place a sheet of nori on a bamboo sushi mat.

2. Spread an even layer of rice over the nori, leaving a margin at the top.

3. Arrange thinly sliced vegetables and avocado down the center of the rice.

4. Roll the sushi tightly using the bamboo mat.

5. Cut the roll into slices and serve with soy sauce.

Prep Time: 30 minutes

Total Time: 30 minutes

Customization: Experiment with different fillings like tofu, mango, or pickled radish.

Mediterranean Couscous Salad

Ingredients:

- Couscous
- Cherry tomatoes
- Cucumber
- Red onion
- Kalamata olives
- Feta cheese
- Fresh parsley
- Lemon juice
- Olive oil
- Salt and pepper

Instructions:

1. Cook couscous according to package instructions and let it cool.
2. Chop tomatoes, cucumber, red onion, and parsley.
3. Mix the cooked couscous with the chopped vegetables, olives, and crumbled feta cheese.
4. Dress with lemon juice, olive oil, salt, and pepper.
5. Toss well and serve chilled.

Prep Time: 15 minutes

Cook Time: 10 minutes

Total Time: 25 minutes

Customization: Add chickpeas or grilled chicken for extra protein.

Spaghetti with Sun-dried Tomato Pesto

Ingredients:

- Spaghetti
- Sun-dried tomatoes
- Garlic
- Pine nuts
- Fresh basil
- Parmesan cheese
- Olive oil
- Salt and pepper

Instructions:

0. Prepare spaghetti as per the instructions on the package.

1. Using a food processor, blend sun-dried tomatoes, garlic, pine nuts, basil, and Parmesan cheese until a smooth mixture forms.

2. Gradually add olive oil while blending until the desired consistency is achieved.

3. Combine the cooked spaghetti with the sun-dried tomato pesto.

4. Season with salt and pepper to your preference before serving.

Prep Time: 10 minutes

Cook Time: 10 minutes

Total Time: 20 minutes

Customization: Add grilled vegetables or shrimp for an extra twist.

Butternut Squash and Sage Risotto

Ingredients:

- Arborio rice
- Butternut squash
- Onion
- Garlic
- Fresh sage
- Vegetable broth
- White wine
- Parmesan cheese
- Butter
- Salt and pepper

Instructions:

1. Peel and dice butternut squash, then roast until tender.
2. In a separate pan, sauté onion, garlic, and fresh sage until fragrant.
3. Add Arborio rice and toast for a few minutes.
4. Gradually add vegetable broth and white wine, stirring constantly until rice is cooked.
5. Stir in roasted butternut squash, Parmesan cheese, and butter until creamy.
6. Season with salt and pepper, garnish with fresh sage, and serve.

Prep Time: 20 minutes

Cook Time: 30 minutes

Total Time: 50 minutes

Customization: Add spinach or kale for extra greens.

Potato and Leek Soup

Ingredients:

- Potatoes
- Leeks
- Vegetable broth
- Garlic
- Thyme
- Heavy cream (optional)

- Salt and pepper

Instructions:

1. Sauté sliced leeks and minced garlic until softened.
2. Add diced potatoes, thyme, and vegetable broth.
3. Simmer until potatoes are tender.
4. Blend until smooth, then stir in heavy cream if desired.
5. Season with salt and pepper, and serve hot.

Prep Time: 10 minutes

Cook Time: 30 minutes

Total Time: 40 minutes

Customization: Add bacon bits or crispy fried shallots for extra flavor and texture.

Thai Mango Salad

Ingredients:

- Ripe mango
- Red bell pepper
- Red onion
- Fresh cilantro
- Mint leaves
- Peanuts
- Lime juice
- Fish sauce
- Sugar
- Chili flakes

Instructions:

1. Julienne mango, red bell pepper, and red onion.
2. Chop fresh cilantro and mint leaves.
3. Toss together with peanuts in a large bowl.
4. Whisk lime juice, fish sauce, sugar, and chili flakes in a small bowl to make the dressing.
5. Pour the dressing over the salad, toss well, and serve.

Prep Time: 15 minutes

Total Time: 15 minutes

Customization: Add cooked shrimp or shredded chicken for added protein.

Falafel Wrap with Tzatziki Sauce

Ingredients:

- Falafel
- Pita bread
- Lettuce
- Tomato
- Cucumber
- Red onion
- Tzatziki sauce

Instructions:

1. Cook falafel according to package instructions.
2. Warm pita bread and spread tzatziki sauce on one side.

3. Fill with falafel, lettuce, tomato, cucumber, and red onion.
4. Roll up tightly and serve.

Prep Time: 10 minutes

Cook Time: 10 minutes

Total Time: 20 minutes

Customization: Add hummus or pickled vegetables for extra flavor.

Pasta Primavera with Spring Vegetables

Ingredients:

- Pasta
- Assorted spring vegetables (such as asparagus, peas, carrots, cherry tomatoes)
- Garlic
- Olive oil
- Lemon zest
- Fresh basil
- Parmesan cheese
- Salt and pepper

Instructions:

1. Cook pasta according to package instructions.
2. Sauté minced garlic in olive oil until fragrant.
3. Add chopped spring vegetables and cook until tender-crisp.
4. Toss cooked pasta with the vegetables, lemon zest, fresh basil, and Parmesan cheese.

5. Season with salt and pepper, and serve hot.

Prep Time: 15 minutes

Cook Time: 15 minutes

Total Time: 30 minutes

Customization: Add grilled chicken or shrimp for extra protein.

Sweet Corn and Zucchini Pie

Ingredients:

- Pie crust
- Sweet corn kernels
- Zucchini
- Onion
- Garlic
- Eggs
- Milk
- Shredded cheese
- Fresh herbs (such as basil or thyme)
- Salt and pepper

Instructions:

1. Preheat oven and blind-bake pie crust according to package instructions.
2. Sauté chopped zucchini, onion, and garlic until softened.
3. In a bowl, whisk together eggs, milk, shredded cheese, fresh herbs, salt, and pepper.

4. Stir in sautéed vegetables and sweet corn kernels.
5. Pour mixture into the pre-baked pie crust and bake until set and golden brown.
6. Allow to cool slightly before slicing and serving.

Prep Time: 20 minutes

Cook Time: 45 minutes

Total Time: 65 minutes

Customization: Add cooked bacon or diced ham for a meaty version.

Grilled Vegetable and Hummus Tart

Ingredients:

- Puff pastry
- Assorted grilled vegetables (such as zucchini, bell peppers, eggplant)
- Hummus
- Fresh herbs (such as parsley or basil)
- Olive oil
- Salt and pepper

Instructions:

- Preheat oven and roll out puff pastry into a rectangle.
- Spread a layer of hummus over the pastry, leaving a border around the edges.
- Arrange grilled vegetables over the hummus.
- Drizzle with olive oil, sprinkle with fresh herbs, salt, and pepper.
- Bake until pastry is golden brown and crisp.
- Allow to cool slightly before slicing and serving.

Prep Time: 15 minutes

Cook Time: 25 minutes

Total Time: 40 minutes

Customization: Add crumbled feta cheese or sliced olives for extra flavor.

Asian Noodle Salad with Peanut Dressing

Ingredients:

- Asian noodles (such as soba or rice noodles)
- Mixed vegetables (such as bell peppers, carrots, cabbage)
- Edamame
- Green onions
- Fresh cilantro
- Peanuts
- Peanut butter
- Soy sauce
- Rice vinegar
- Sesame oil
- Honey
- Garlic
- Ginger

- Lime juice
- Red pepper flakes

Instructions:

1. Cook noodles according to package instructions, then rinse under cold water and drain well.
2. Prep vegetables by julienning or chopping into bite-sized pieces.
3. In a large bowl, combine cooked noodles, mixed vegetables, edamame, chopped green onions, chopped cilantro, and peanuts.
4. In a separate bowl, whisk together peanut butter, soy sauce, rice vinegar, sesame oil, honey, minced garlic, minced ginger, lime juice, and red pepper flakes to make the dressing.
5. Pour the dressing over the salad and toss until well combined.
6. Serve chilled or at room temperature.

Prep Time: 20 minutes

Cook Time: 10 minutes

Total Time: 30 minutes

Customization: Add cooked chicken, tofu, or shrimp for additional protein.

Roasted Beet and Citrus Salad

Ingredients:

- Beets
- Mixed greens
- Oranges
- Grapefruit
- Goat cheese
- Walnuts
- Balsamic vinegar
- Olive oil
- Honey
- Dijon mustard
- Salt and pepper

Instructions:

1. Preheat oven and roast beets until tender, then peel and slice.
2. Segment oranges and grapefruit, reserving any juices.
3. Arrange mixed greens on a serving platter and top with roasted beets, citrus segments, crumbled goat cheese, and chopped walnuts.
4. In a small bowl, whisk together balsamic vinegar, olive oil, honey, Dijon mustard, salt, and pepper to make the dressing, adding reserved citrus juices if desired.
5. Drizzle the dressing over the salad and serve.

Prep Time: 15 minutes

Cook Time: 45 minutes

Total Time: 60 minutes

Customization: Add cooked quinoa or grilled chicken for extra protein.

These lunch recipes offer a wide range of flavors and ingredients to suit various tastes and dietary preferences.

Dinner Recipes

Potato Gnocchi with Tomato Basil Sauce

Ingredients:

- Potato gnocchi
- Olive oil
- Garlic
- Canned tomatoes
- Fresh basil
- Salt and pepper
- Grated Parmesan cheese (optional)

Instructions:

1. Cook potato gnocchi according to package instructions.
2. In a separate pan, heat olive oil and sauté minced garlic until fragrant.
3. Add canned tomatoes and simmer until slightly thickened.
4. Stir in chopped fresh basil and season with salt and pepper to taste.
5. Toss cooked gnocchi in the tomato basil sauce until well coated.
6. Serve hot with grated Parmesan cheese if desired.

Prep Time: 10 minutes

Cook Time: 20 minutes

Total Time: 30 minutes

Customization: Add cooked Italian sausage or sautéed vegetables for extra flavor and nutrients.

Creamy Polenta with Roasted Mushrooms

Ingredients:

- Cornmeal
- Vegetable broth
- Butter
- Parmesan cheese
- Mushrooms
- Olive oil
- Garlic
- Thyme
- Salt and pepper

Instructions:

1. In a saucepan, bring vegetable broth to a boil.
2. Gradually whisk in cornmeal and cook until thick and creamy.
3. Stir in butter and grated Parmesan cheese until melted.

4. Meanwhile, toss mushrooms with olive oil, minced garlic, fresh thyme, salt, and pepper.
5. Roast mushrooms in the oven until golden and tender.
6. Serve creamy polenta topped with roasted mushrooms.

Prep Time: 10 minutes

Cook Time: 30 minutes

Total Time: 40 minutes

Customization: Add roasted cherry tomatoes or sautéed spinach for extra color and flavor contrast.

Vegetable Paella

Ingredients

- Arborio rice
- Vegetable broth
- Onion
- Bell peppers
- Tomatoes
- Green beans
- Artichoke hearts
- Garlic
- Saffron threads
- Paprika
- Frozen peas
- Lemon wedges
- Fresh parsley
- Olive oil
- Salt and pepper

Instructions:

1. In a large skillet, sauté diced onion and minced garlic in olive oil until softened.
2. Add chopped bell peppers, diced tomatoes, sliced green beans, and drained artichoke hearts. Cook until vegetables are tender.
3. Stir in Arborio rice, saffron threads, and paprika. Cook for a few minutes until rice is coated.
4. Gradually add vegetable broth, stirring occasionally until rice is cooked and liquid is absorbed.
5. Stir in frozen peas and cook until heated through.
6. Season with salt and pepper, garnish with fresh parsley, and serve with lemon wedges.

Prep Time: 20 minutes

Cook Time: 40 minutes

Total Time: 60 minutes

Customization: Add chickpeas or tofu for extra protein and texture.

Chickpea and Spinach Curry

Ingredients:

- Chickpeas
- Onion
- Garlic
- Ginger
- Tomato puree
- Spinach

-   Coconut milk
-   Curry powder
-   Turmeric
-   Cumin
-   Coriander
-   Cayenne pepper (optional)
-   Lemon juice
-   Olive oil
-   Salt and pepper

Instructions:

1. Sauté diced onion, minced garlic, and grated ginger in olive oil until softened.
2. Add tomato puree, curry powder, turmeric, cumin, coriander, and cayenne pepper. Cook for a few minutes until fragrant.
3. Stir in drained chickpeas and coconut milk. Simmer until chickpeas are heated through.
4. Add fresh spinach and cook until wilted.
5. Season with lemon juice, salt, and pepper to taste.
6. Serve hot with rice or naan bread.

Prep Time: 15 minutes

Cook Time: 20 minutes

Total Time: 35 minutes

Customization: Add diced tomatoes or bell peppers for extra texture and flavor.

Lentil and Sweet Potato Shepherd's Pie

Ingredients:

-   Lentils
-   Sweet potatoes
-   Onion
-   Carrots
-   Celery
-   Garlic
-   Vegetable broth
-   Tomato paste
-   Worcestershire sauce (optional)
-   Fresh thyme
-   Olive oil
-   Salt and pepper

Instructions:

1. Cook lentils according to package instructions until tender.
2. Meanwhile, peel and dice sweet potatoes, then boil until soft.
3. Sauté diced onion, carrots, celery, and minced garlic in olive oil until softened.
4. Add cooked lentils, tomato paste, Worcestershire sauce, fresh thyme, salt, and pepper. Cook until flavors are blended.
5. Mash boiled sweet potatoes with a bit of olive oil until smooth.
6. Transfer lentil mixture to a baking dish and spread mashed sweet potatoes over the top.
7. Bake in the oven until bubbly and golden brown.

Prep Time: 20 minutes

Cook Time: 40 minutes

Total Time: 60 minutes

Customization: Add peas or corn to the lentil mixture for extra sweetness and color.

Stuffed Acorn Squash with Quinoa and Cranberries

Ingredients:

- Acorn squash
- Quinoa
- Vegetable broth
- Onion
- Celery
- Dried cranberries
- Pecans
- Fresh parsley
- Maple syrup
- Cinnamon
- Nutmeg
- Olive oil
- Salt and pepper

Instructions:

1. Preheat oven and halve acorn squash, removing seeds.
2. Brush cut sides with olive oil and season with salt and pepper.
3. Roast squash halves in the oven until tender.
4. Cook quinoa in vegetable broth until fluffy.
5. Meanwhile, sauté diced onion and celery in olive oil until softened.
6. Stir cooked quinoa, dried cranberries, chopped pecans, fresh parsley, maple syrup, cinnamon, and nutmeg into the sautéed vegetables.
7. Spoon quinoa mixture into roasted acorn squash halves.
8. Return stuffed squash to the oven and bake until heated through.

Prep Time: 20 minutes

Cook Time: 45 minutes

Total Time: 65 minutes

Customization: Add diced apple or raisins for extra sweetness and texture.

Mushroom and Barley Pilaf

Ingredients:

- Pearl barley
- Vegetable broth
- Mushrooms
- Onion
- Garlic
- Thyme
- Parsley
- Olive oil
- Butter
- Salt and pepper

Instructions:

1. Cook pearl barley in vegetable broth until tender.
2. Meanwhile, sauté sliced mushrooms, diced onion, and minced garlic in olive oil and butter until golden.
3. Stir cooked barley into the mushroom mixture.
4. Season with fresh thyme, chopped parsley, salt, and pepper to taste.
5. Serve hot as a hearty and flavorful side dish.

Prep Time: 10 minutes

Cook Time: 40 minutes

Total Time: 50 minutes

Customization: Add chopped spinach or kale for extra greens and nutrients.

Pumpkin Lasagna

Ingredients:

- Lasagna noodles
- Pumpkin puree
- Ricotta cheese
- Mozzarella cheese
- Parmesan cheese
- Egg
- Garlic
- Sage
- Nutmeg
- Salt and pepper
- Marinara sauce

Instructions:

1. Cook lasagna noodles according to package instructions until al dente.
2. In a bowl, mix pumpkin puree, ricotta cheese, grated mozzarella cheese, grated Parmesan cheese, beaten egg, minced garlic, chopped sage, nutmeg, salt, and pepper.
3. Spread a layer of marinara sauce in a baking dish.
4. Layer cooked lasagna noodles, pumpkin mixture, and marinara sauce.
5. Repeat layers until all ingredients are used, ending with marinara sauce on top.
6. Sprinkle with extra mozzarella and Parmesan cheese.
7. Bake in the oven until bubbly and golden brown.

Prep Time: 30 minutes

Cook Time: 45 minutes

Total Time: 75 minutes

Customization: Add cooked ground meat or sautéed vegetables for extra protein and flavor.

Teriyaki Tofu with Sticky Rice

Ingredients:

- Firm tofu
- Soy sauce
- Mirin
- Brown sugar
- Garlic
- Ginger
- Cornstarch
- Sticky rice
- Sesame seeds
- Green onions
- Olive oil
- Salt and pepper

Instructions:

1. Press tofu to remove excess moisture, then cut into cubes.
2. In a bowl, whisk together soy sauce, mirin, brown sugar, minced garlic, grated ginger, and cornstarch to make the teriyaki sauce.
3. Sauté tofu cubes in olive oil until golden and crispy.
4. Pour teriyaki sauce over tofu and simmer until thickened.
5. Cook sticky rice according to package instructions.
6. Serve teriyaki tofu over sticky rice, garnished with sesame seeds and chopped green onions.

Prep Time: 20 minutes

Cook Time: 30 minutes

Total Time: 50 minutes

Customization: Add stir-fried vegetables like bell peppers, broccoli, or snap peas for extra color and nutrients.

Moroccan Vegetable Tagine

Ingredients:

- Carrots
- Potatoes
- Eggplant
- Zucchini
- Bell peppers
- Onion
- Garlic
- Tomato paste
- Vegetable broth
- Chickpeas
- Dried apricots
- Almonds
- Ras el hanout (Moroccan spice blend)
- Cinnamon
- Olive oil
- Salt and pepper

- **Instructions:**

1. Sauté diced onion and minced garlic in olive oil until softened.
2. Add diced carrots, potatoes, eggplant, zucchini, and bell peppers. Cook until slightly caramelized.
3. Stir in tomato paste, ras el hanout, cinnamon, salt, and pepper.

4. Add vegetable broth and simmer until vegetables are tender.
5. Stir in drained chickpeas, chopped dried apricots, and sliced almonds.
6. Serve hot as a flavorful and aromatic stew.

- **Prep Time:** 20 minutes

- **Cook Time:** 40 minutes

- **Total Time:** 60 minutes

- **Customization:** Add couscous or quinoa as a side dish to soak up the delicious sauce.

Spicy Black Bean Tacos

Ingredients:

- Black beans
- Onion
- Garlic
- Jalapeño
- Cumin
- Chili powder
- Paprika
- Cayenne pepper
- Lime juice
- Corn tortillas
- Avocado
- Cilantro
- Salsa
- Lime wedges
- Olive oil
- Salt and pepper

Instructions:

1. Sauté diced onion, minced garlic, and chopped jalapeño in olive oil until softened.
2. Add drained black beans, cumin, chili powder, paprika, cayenne pepper, and lime juice. Cook until heated through.
3. Warm corn tortillas in a dry skillet until soft and pliable.
4. Spoon black bean mixture into tortillas and top with sliced avocado, chopped cilantro, and salsa.
5. Serve hot with lime wedges for squeezing.

Prep Time: 15 minutes

Cook Time: 15 minutes

Total Time: 30 minutes

Customization: Add shredded lettuce or cabbage for extra crunch and freshness.

Corn Chowder with Bell Peppers

Ingredients:

- Corn kernels
- Bell peppers
- Onion
- Garlic
- Potatoes
- Vegetable broth

- Heavy cream
- Thyme
- Smoked paprika
- Cayenne pepper
- Olive oil
- Salt and pepper

Instructions:

1. Sauté diced onion and minced garlic in olive oil until softened.
2. Add diced bell peppers and cook until slightly caramelized.
3. Stir in corn kernels and diced potatoes.
4. Add vegetable broth, thyme, smoked paprika, cayenne pepper, salt, and pepper.
5. Simmer until potatoes are tender.
6. Stir in heavy cream and cook until heated through.
7. Serve hot as a comforting and creamy soup.

Prep Time: 20 minutes

Cook Time: 30 minutes

Total Time: 50 minutes

Customization: Add diced bacon or ham for extra richness and flavor.

Zucchini and Tomato Tart

Ingredients:

- Puff pastry
- Zucchini
- Tomatoes
- Onion
- Garlic
- Fresh basil
- Parmesan cheese
- Olive oil
- Balsamic glaze
- Salt and pepper

Instructions:

1. Preheat oven and roll out puff pastry into a rectangle.
2. Score a border around the pastry and prick the center with a fork.
3. Spread a layer of caramelized onion and minced garlic over the center of the pastry.
4. Arrange thinly sliced zucchini and tomatoes over the onion mixture.
5. Drizzle with olive oil, sprinkle with grated Parmesan cheese, salt, and pepper.
6. Bake in the oven until pastry is golden brown and vegetables are tender.
7. Garnish with fresh basil and a drizzle of balsamic glaze before serving.

Prep Time: 20 minutes

Cook Time: 25 minutes

Total Time: 45 minutes

Customization: Add sliced mushrooms or bell peppers for extra variety and flavor.

Eggplant Parmesan

Ingredients:

- Eggplant
- Eggs
- Breadcrumbs
- Parmesan cheese
- Marinara sauce
- Mozzarella cheese
- Olive oil
- Fresh basil
- Salt and pepper

Instructions:

1. Preheat oven and slice eggplant into rounds.
2. Dip eggplant slices in beaten eggs, then coat with breadcrumbs mixed with grated Parmesan cheese.
3. Heat olive oil in a skillet and fry breaded eggplant slices until golden brown on both sides.
4. Spread a layer of marinara sauce in a baking dish.
5. Arrange fried eggplant slices in the dish, overlapping slightly.
6. Top with more marinara sauce and grated mozzarella cheese.
7. Bake in the oven until cheese is melted and bubbly.
8. Garnish with fresh basil before serving.

Prep Time: 20 minutes

Cook Time: 40 minutes

Total Time: 60 minutes

Customization: Add a layer of sautéed spinach or mushrooms between the eggplant slices for extra flavor and nutrients.

Rice and Bean Stuffed Peppers

Ingredients:

- Bell peppers
- Rice
- Black beans
- Onion
- Garlic
- Tomato sauce
- Chili powder
- Cumin
- Paprika
- Cilantro
- Lime juice
- Olive oil
- Salt and pepper

Instructions:

1. Preheat oven and halve bell peppers, removing seeds and membranes.
2. Cook rice according to package instructions until fluffy.

3. Meanwhile, sauté diced onion and minced garlic in olive oil until softened.
4. Stir in cooked rice, drained black beans, tomato sauce, chili powder, cumin, paprika, chopped cilantro, lime juice, salt, and pepper.
5. Fill bell pepper halves with the rice and bean mixture.
6. Bake in the oven until peppers are tender and filling is heated through.
7. Serve hot as a satisfying and nutritious meal.

Prep Time: 20 minutes

Cook Time: 30 minutes

Total Time: 50 minutes

Customization: Add diced tomatoes or corn to the rice and bean mixture for extra texture and flavor.

Snack Recipes
Energy Balls with Oats and Dates

Ingredients:

- Rolled oats
- Dates
- Almond butter
- Honey
- Chia seeds
- Vanilla extract
- Coconut flakes (optional)

Instructions:

1. In a food processor, blend rolled oats until they form a coarse flour-like texture.
2. Add pitted dates, almond butter, honey, chia seeds, and vanilla extract to the food processor. Pulse until well combined and the mixture sticks together.
3. If desired, roll the mixture into small balls and coat with coconut flakes.
4. Refrigerate for at least 30 minutes before serving.

Prep Time: 15 minutes

Total Time: 45 minutes

Customization: Add cocoa powder for chocolate flavor, or swap almond butter for peanut butter for a different taste.

Homemade Banana Bread

Ingredients:

- Ripe bananas
- All-purpose flour
- Baking powder
- Baking soda
- Salt
- Unsalted butter
- Brown sugar
- Eggs

- Vanilla extract

Instructions:

1. Preheat oven and grease a loaf pan.
2. In a bowl, mash ripe bananas until smooth.
3. In a separate bowl, whisk together flour, baking powder, baking soda, and salt.
4. Cream softened butter and brown sugar until light and fluffy. Beat in eggs one at a time, then stir in vanilla extract.
5. Gradually mix in dry ingredients until just incorporated, then fold in mashed bananas.
6. Pour batter into the prepared loaf pan and bake until golden brown and a toothpick inserted into the center comes out clean.
7. Allow to cool before slicing and serving.

Prep Time: 15 minutes

Cook Time: 60 minutes

Total Time: 75 minutes

Customization: Add nuts or chocolate chips to the batter for added texture and flavor.

Apple Chips

Ingredients:

- Apples
- Cinnamon
- Sugar (optional)

Instructions:

1. Preheat oven and line baking sheets with parchment paper.
2. Slice apples thinly using a sharp knife or mandoline slicer.
3. Arrange apple slices in a single layer on the prepared baking sheets.
4. Sprinkle with cinnamon and sugar if desired.
5. Bake in the oven until crisp, flipping halfway through.
6. Allow to cool before serving.

Prep Time: 10 minutes

Cook Time: 90 minutes

Total Time: 100 minutes

Customization: Try using different spices like nutmeg or pumpkin pie spice for variation.

Cinnamon Sugar Pretzels

Ingredients:

- Pretzels
- Butter
- Cinnamon
- Sugar

Instructions:

1. Preheat oven and line a baking sheet with parchment paper.
2. Melt butter in a microwave-safe bowl.
3. In a separate bowl, mix together cinnamon and sugar.
4. Dip pretzels in melted butter, then roll in the cinnamon sugar mixture until coated.
5. Place coated pretzels on the prepared baking sheet.
6. Bake in the oven until golden and crispy.
7. Allow to cool before serving.

Prep Time: 10 minutes

Cook Time: 15 minutes

Total Time: 25 minutes

Customization: Add a pinch of nutmeg or ginger to the cinnamon sugar mixture for extra flavor.

Trail Mix with Dried Fruit and Nuts

Ingredients:

- Assorted nuts (such as almonds, cashews, peanuts)
- Dried fruit (such as raisins, cranberries, apricots)
- Chocolate chips (optional)

Instructions:

1. Mix together assorted nuts, dried fruit, and chocolate chips in a large bowl.
2. Store in an airtight container for snacking on the go.

Prep Time: 5 minutes

Total Time: 5 minutes

Customization: Customize the mix with your favorite nuts, fruits, and chocolates.

Peanut Butter and Jelly Smoothie

Ingredients:

- Banana
- Frozen berries (such as strawberries, blueberries)
- Peanut butter
- Greek yogurt
- Milk (or almond milk)
- Honey (optional)

Instructions:

1. Combine banana, frozen berries, peanut butter, Greek yogurt, milk, and honey in a blender.
2. Blend until smooth and creamy.
3. Pour into glasses and serve immediately.

Prep Time: 5 minutes

Total Time: 5 minutes

Customization: Use almond butter or other nut butters for a different flavor profile.

Yogurt with Honey and Walnuts

Ingredients:

- Greek yogurt
- Honey
- Walnuts (or other nuts)

Instructions:

1. Spoon Greek yogurt into serving bowls.
2. Drizzle with honey and sprinkle with chopped walnuts.
3. Serve immediately as a simple and nutritious snack.

Prep Time: 2 minutes

Total Time: 2 minutes

Customization: Add fresh fruit or granola for extra flavor and texture.

Baked Sweet Potato Fries

Ingredients:

- Sweet potatoes
- Olive oil
- Salt and pepper

Instructions:

1. Preheat oven and line a baking sheet with parchment paper.
2. Peel sweet potatoes and cut into fries.
3. Toss sweet potato fries with olive oil, salt, and pepper until evenly coated.
4. Arrange fries in a single layer on the prepared baking sheet.
5. Bake in the oven until crispy and golden brown, flipping halfway through.
6. Serve hot with your favorite dipping sauce.

Prep Time: 10 minutes

Cook Time: 30 minutes

Total Time: 40 minutes

Customization: Sprinkle with smoked paprika or chili powder for a spicy kick.

Fruit Salsa with Cinnamon Tortilla Chips

Ingredients:

- Assorted fruits (such as strawberries, kiwi, pineapple, mango)
- Lime juice
- Honey
- Cinnamon
- Flour tortillas
- Olive oil spray

1. Chop assorted fruits into small pieces and toss with lime juice and honey.
2. Sprinkle with cinnamon and stir to combine.
3. Preheat oven and cut flour tortillas into wedges.
4. Arrange tortilla wedges on a baking sheet and spray with olive oil.
5. Sprinkle with cinnamon and bake until crispy.
6. Serve fruit salsa with cinnamon tortilla chips for a refreshing and crunchy snack.

Prep Time: 15 minutes

Cook Time: 10 minutes

Total Time: 25 minutes

Customization: Use different fruits according to your preference and seasonal availability.

Ricotta and Honey Bruschetta

Ingredients:

- Baguette
- Ricotta cheese
- Honey
- Fresh basil
- Olive oil
- Salt and pepper

Instructions:

1. Preheat oven and slice baguette into rounds.
2. Drizzle baguette slices with olive oil and sprinkle with salt and pepper.
3. Toast baguette slices in the oven until crispy and golden brown.
4. Spread ricotta cheese on toasted baguette slices.
5. Drizzle with honey and garnish with fresh basil leaves.
6. Serve immediately as a sweet and savory appetizer or snack.

Prep Time: 10 minutes

Cook Time: 10 minutes

Total Time: 20 minutes

Customization: Add sliced figs or strawberries on top for extra sweetness and flavor.

Must Read!!!

Thank you for choosing to explore my book! Your support means the world to me. As a valued reader, your review holds immense significance. Your insights not only guide potential readers but also contribute to shaping the ongoing journey of this book. Your thoughts help in fostering a community of engaged readers, making the experience richer for everyone.

How You Can Share Your Review?

Sharing your review on Amazon allows others to benefit from your perspective, aiding them in their decision-making process.

To post your review, simply visit the Amazon page where you discovered my book, head to the 'Customer Reviews' section, and click on 'Write a customer review' to share your invaluable feedback.

Alternatively, you can effortlessly access the review section by scanning the QR code below with your smartphone. Thank you once again for your support and for considering sharing your thoughts with us.

Chapter 6: Low Carb Day Recipes

Breakfast Recipes

Avocado and Egg Breakfast Bowl

Ingredients:

- Avocado
- Eggs
- Salt and pepper
- Optional toppings: cherry tomatoes, feta cheese, salsa

Instructions:

1. Slice the avocado in half and remove the pit.
2. Scoop out a bit of avocado flesh to make room for the egg.
3. Crack an egg into each avocado half.
4. Season with salt and pepper.
5. Bake in the oven until the eggs are cooked to your desired doneness.

6. Top with optional toppings like cherry tomatoes, feta cheese, or salsa.

Prep Time: 5 minutes

Cook Time: 15 minutes

Total Time: 20 minutes

Customization: Add cooked bacon or smoked salmon for extra flavor and protein.

Spinach and Mushroom Omelette

Ingredients:

- Eggs
- Spinach
- Mushrooms
- Olive oil
- Salt and pepper
- Optional: cheese, diced tomatoes, onions

Instructions:

1. Heat olive oil in a skillet over medium heat.
2. Sauté sliced mushrooms until golden brown.
3. Add fresh spinach to the skillet and cook until wilted.
4. Whisk eggs in a bowl and pour over the spinach and mushrooms.
5. Cook until the eggs are set, then fold the omelette in half.
6. Season with salt and pepper.

7. Top with optional ingredients like cheese, diced tomatoes, or onions.

Prep Time: 5 minutes

Cook Time: 10 minutes

Total Time: 15 minutes

Customization: Use your favorite vegetables or herbs for filling, such as bell peppers or basil.

Greek Yogurt with Nuts and Seeds

Ingredients:

- Greek yogurt
- Mixed nuts (such as almonds, walnuts, pecans)
- Seeds (such as chia seeds, pumpkin seeds)
- Honey (optional)

Instructions:

1. Spoon Greek yogurt into a bowl.
2. Sprinkle with mixed nuts and seeds.
3. Drizzle with honey if desired.

Prep Time: 2 minutes

Total Time: 2 minutes

Customization: Add fresh berries or sliced fruits for extra sweetness and flavor.

Smoked Salmon and Cream Cheese Roll-Ups

Ingredients:

- Smoked salmon
- Cream cheese
- Cucumber (optional)
- Chives (optional)

Instructions:

1. Lay out slices of smoked salmon on a clean surface.
2. Spread a thin layer of cream cheese over each slice.
3. If desired, add a slice of cucumber or sprinkle with chopped chives.
4. Roll up each slice tightly.

Prep Time: 5 minutes

Total Time: 5 minutes

Customization: Add avocado slices or capers for extra flavor and texture.

Cauliflower Hash Browns

Ingredients:

- Cauliflower
- Eggs
- Almond flour
- Garlic powder
- Salt and pepper
- Olive oil

Instructions:

1. Grate cauliflower using a box grater or food processor.
2. Squeeze out excess moisture from the cauliflower using a clean kitchen towel.
3. In a bowl, mix together grated cauliflower, eggs, almond flour, garlic powder, salt, and pepper.
4. Form the mixture into patties.
5. Heat olive oil in a skillet over medium heat.
6. Cook the cauliflower patties until golden brown on both sides.

Prep Time: 15 minutes

Cook Time: 10 minutes

Total Time: 25 minutes

Customization: Add shredded cheese or herbs to the cauliflower mixture for extra flavor.

Almond Flour Pancakes

Ingredients:

- Almond flour
- Eggs
- Baking powder
- Salt
- Unsweetened almond milk
- Vanilla extract

- Optional: berries, sugar-free syrup

Instructions:

1. In a bowl, whisk together almond flour, eggs, baking powder, salt, almond milk, and vanilla extract until smooth.
2. Heat a non-stick skillet over medium heat and grease lightly.
3. Pour batter onto the skillet to form pancakes.
4. Cook until bubbles form on the surface, then flip and cook until golden brown.
5. Serve with optional toppings like fresh berries or sugar-free syrup.

Prep Time: 5 minutes

Cook Time: 10 minutes

Total Time: 15 minutes

Customization: Add cinnamon or nutmeg to the batter for extra flavor.

Coconut and Chia Seed Pudding

Ingredients:

- Coconut milk
- Chia seeds
- Vanilla extract
- Sweetener of choice (such as stevia, erythritol)
- Optional toppings: berries, shredded coconut, nuts

Instructions:

1. In a bowl, mix together coconut milk, chia seeds, vanilla extract, and sweetener.
2. Stir well to combine, then cover and refrigerate overnight.
3. Serve chilled with optional toppings like berries, shredded coconut, or nuts.

Prep Time: 5 minutes

Total Time: 5 minutes (+ overnight refrigeration)

Customization: Use different types of milk (such as almond milk) or flavorings (such as cocoa powder) for variation.

Turkey and Spinach Scrambled Eggs

Ingredients:

- Eggs
- Turkey slices (or ground turkey)
- Fresh spinach
- Salt and pepper
- Olive oil

Instructions:

1. Heat olive oil in a skillet over medium heat.
2. Add turkey slices (or ground turkey) and cook until browned.
3. Add fresh spinach to the skillet and cook until wilted.

4. Whisk eggs in a bowl and pour over the turkey and spinach.
5. Cook until the eggs are scrambled and fully cooked.
6. Season with salt and pepper.

Prep Time: 5 minutes

Cook Time: 10 minutes

Total Time: 15 minutes

Customization: Add diced tomatoes or onions for extra flavor.

Bacon and Egg Muffins

Ingredients:

- Bacon slices
- Eggs
- Salt and pepper
- Optional: shredded cheese, diced vegetables

Instructions:

1. Preheat oven and grease a muffin tin.
2. Line each muffin cup with a slice of bacon, creating a cup shape.
3. Crack an egg into each bacon-lined muffin cup.
4. Season with salt and pepper.
5. Bake in the oven until the eggs are set.
6. Remove from the oven and let cool slightly before serving.

Prep Time: 10 minutes

Cook Time: 20 minutes

Total Time: 30 minutes

Customization: Add shredded cheese or diced vegetables to each muffin cup before cracking the egg for extra flavor and nutrients.

Sautéed Greens with Garlic and Olive Oil

Ingredients:

- Mixed greens (such as kale, spinach, Swiss chard)
- Garlic
- Olive oil
- Salt and pepper

Instructions:

1. Heat olive oil in a skillet over medium heat.
2. Add minced garlic to the skillet and sauté until fragrant.
3. Add mixed greens to the skillet and cook until wilted.
4. Season with salt and pepper to taste.
5. Serve hot as a nutritious side dish or base for other breakfast items.

Prep Time: 5 minutes

Cook Time: 5 minutes

Total Time: 10 minutes

Customization: Add red pepper flakes for a spicy kick, or finish with a squeeze of lemon juice for brightness.

Cheese and Herb Frittata

Ingredients:

- Eggs
- Cheese (such as cheddar, feta)
- Fresh herbs (such as parsley, chives)
- Salt and pepper
- Olive oil

Instructions:

1. Preheat oven and grease a baking dish.
2. Whisk eggs in a bowl and stir in grated cheese and chopped fresh herbs.
3. Season with salt and pepper.
4. Pour the egg mixture into the prepared baking dish.
5. Bake in the oven until the frittata is set and golden brown on top.
6. Slice and serve hot or cold.

Prep Time: 10 minutes

Cook Time: 20 minutes

Total Time: 30 minutes

Customization: Add diced vegetables like bell peppers or mushrooms for extra flavor and texture.

Protein Smoothie with Avocado and Cocoa

Ingredients:

- Avocado
- Protein powder (such as whey or plant-based)
- Unsweetened cocoa powder
- Unsweetened almond milk
- Optional: spinach, banana, sweetener of choice

Instructions:

1. Combine avocado, protein powder, cocoa powder, and almond milk in a blender.
2. Blend until smooth and creamy.
3. Add optional ingredients like spinach, banana, or sweetener if desired.
4. Blend again until well combined.
5. Pour into glasses and serve immediately.

Prep Time: 5 minutes

Total Time: 5 minutes

Customization: Add a tablespoon of nut butter for extra creaminess and flavor, or top with shredded coconut or chopped nuts for texture.

Lunch Recipes

Chicken Caesar Salad (no croutons)

Ingredients:

- Chicken breast
- Romaine lettuce
- Caesar dressing (without added sugar)
- Parmesan cheese
- Olive oil
- Salt and pepper

Instructions:

1. Season chicken breast with salt and pepper, then grill or bake until cooked through.
2. Chop romaine lettuce and place it in a large bowl.
3. Slice cooked chicken breast and add it to the bowl.
4. Drizzle with Caesar dressing and toss to coat evenly.
5. Top with shaved Parmesan cheese.

Prep Time: 10 minutes

Cook Time: 15 minutes

Total Time: 25 minutes

Customization: Add cherry tomatoes, avocado slices, or crispy bacon for extra flavor.

Zucchini Noodle Salad with Pesto

Ingredients:

- Zucchini
- Cherry tomatoes
- Basil pesto
- Pine nuts
- Parmesan cheese
- Olive oil
- Salt and pepper

Instructions:

1. Use a spiralizer to make zucchini noodles (zoodles).
2. Halve cherry tomatoes and add them to the zoodles in a bowl.
3. Toss with basil pesto until evenly coated.
4. Toast pine nuts in a dry skillet until golden brown.
5. Sprinkle toasted pine nuts and shaved Parmesan cheese over the salad.
6. Drizzle with olive oil and season with salt and pepper to taste.

Prep Time: 10 minutes

Total Time: 10 minutes

Customization: Add grilled chicken or shrimp for added protein.

Shrimp and Avocado Salad

Ingredients:

- Shrimp
- Avocado
- Mixed greens
- Cherry tomatoes
- Red onion
- Cilantro
- Lime juice
- Olive oil
- Salt and pepper

Instructions:

1. Cook shrimp in a skillet with olive oil until pink and opaque.
2. Slice avocado and halve cherry tomatoes.
3. Arrange mixed greens on a plate and top with cooked shrimp, avocado slices, cherry tomatoes, thinly sliced red onion, and chopped cilantro.
4. Drizzle with lime juice and olive oil.
5. Season with salt and pepper to taste.

Prep Time: 10 minutes

Cook Time: 5 minutes

Total Time: 15 minutes

Customization: Add cucumber slices or bell peppers for extra crunch.

Stuffed Bell Peppers with Ground Turkey

Ingredients:

- Bell peppers
- Ground turkey
- Onion
- Garlic
- Tomato sauce
- Italian seasoning
- Mozzarella cheese
- Olive oil
- Salt and pepper

Instructions:

1. Preheat oven and cut the tops off bell peppers, removing seeds and membranes.
2. Sauté diced onion and minced garlic in olive oil until softened.
3. Add ground turkey to the skillet and cook until browned.
4. Stir in tomato sauce and Italian seasoning, and season with salt and pepper.
5. Spoon the turkey mixture into the hollowed-out bell peppers.
6. Top with shredded mozzarella cheese.
7. Bake in the oven until the peppers are tender and the cheese is melted and bubbly.

Prep Time: 15 minutes

Cook Time: 30 minutes

Total Time: 45 minutes

Customization: Use ground beef or chicken instead of turkey, and add cooked rice or quinoa to the filling for extra texture.

Broccoli and Stilton Soup

Ingredients:

- Broccoli
- Stilton cheese (or blue cheese)
- Onion
- Garlic
- Vegetable broth
- Heavy cream (optional)
- Olive oil
- Salt and pepper

Instructions:

1. Sauté diced onion and minced garlic in olive oil until softened.
2. Add chopped broccoli florets to the pot and cook until tender.
3. Pour in vegetable broth and simmer until broccoli is very soft.
4. Blend the soup until smooth using an immersion blender or countertop blender.
5. Crumble Stilton cheese into the soup and stir until melted.
6. Stir in heavy cream if using.
7. Season with salt and pepper to taste.

Prep Time: 10 minutes

Cook Time: 20 minutes

Total Time: 30 minutes

Customization: Use other types of cheese like cheddar or Gruyère, and add a sprinkle of nutmeg or thyme for extra flavor.

Tuna Salad Stuffed Avocados

Ingredients:

- Canned tuna
- Avocado
- Celery
- Red onion
- Lemon juice
- Dijon mustard
- Olive oil
- Salt and pepper

Instructions:

1. Drain canned tuna and place it in a bowl.
2. Add diced celery, finely chopped red onion, lemon juice, Dijon mustard, and olive oil to the bowl.
3. Mix well and season with salt and pepper to taste.
4. Cut avocados in half and remove the pits.
5. Spoon tuna salad into the hollowed-out avocado halves.

Prep Time: 10 minutes

Total Time: 10 minutes

Customization: Add chopped pickles or capers for extra flavor and texture.

Eggplant and Tomato Stacks with Feta Cheese

Ingredients:

- Eggplant
- Tomatoes
- Feta cheese
- Fresh basil
- Balsamic vinegar
- Olive oil
- Salt and pepper

Instructions:

1. Slice eggplant and tomatoes into rounds.
2. Brush with olive oil and season with salt and pepper.
3. Grill or roast the eggplant and tomatoes until tender.
4. Stack alternating slices of eggplant and tomato on a plate.
5. Top with crumbled feta cheese and chopped fresh basil.
6. Drizzle with balsamic vinegar and olive oil.

Prep Time: 10 minutes

Cook Time: 15 minutes

Total Time: 25 minutes

Customization: Add grilled chicken or shrimp for added protein.

Beef and Vegetable Stir Fry

Ingredients:

- Beef strips (such as sirloin or flank steak)
- Mixed vegetables (such as bell peppers, broccoli, snap peas)
- Garlic
- Ginger
- Soy sauce (or tamari for gluten-free)
- Sesame oil
- Olive oil
- Salt and pepper

Instructions:

1. Heat olive oil in a skillet or wok over high heat.
2. Add beef strips and stir-fry until browned on all sides.
3. Remove beef from the skillet and set aside.
4. Add more olive oil to the skillet if needed, then stir-fry mixed vegetables until crisp-tender.
5. Add minced garlic and ginger to the skillet and cook until fragrant.
6. Return the beef to the skillet and toss everything together.

7. Drizzle with soy sauce and sesame oil, and season with salt and pepper.

Prep Time: 15 minutes

Cook Time: 10 minutes

Total Time: 25 minutes

Customization: Use chicken or tofu instead of beef, and add chili flakes or Sriracha for heat.

Chicken Lettuce Wraps

Ingredients:

- Ground chicken
- Lettuce leaves (such as iceberg or butter lettuce)
- Onion
- Garlic
- Soy sauce (or tamari for gluten-free)
- Hoisin sauce
- Rice vinegar
- Olive oil
- Green onions
- Salt and pepper

Instructions:

1. Heat olive oil in a skillet over medium heat.
2. Sauté diced onion and minced garlic until softened.
3. Add ground chicken to the skillet and cook until browned.
4. Stir in soy sauce, hoisin sauce, and rice vinegar, and cook until heated through.
5. Season with salt and pepper to taste.
6. Spoon chicken mixture into lettuce leaves and garnish with sliced green onions.

Prep Time: 10 minutes

Cook Time: 10 minutes

Total Time: 20 minutes

Customization: Add diced water chestnuts or mushrooms for extra crunch.

Salmon and Asparagus Bundles

Ingredients:

- Salmon fillets
- Asparagus spears
- Lemon
- Olive oil
- Garlic
- Salt and pepper

Instructions:

1. Preheat oven and line a baking sheet with parchment paper.
2. Season salmon fillets with salt, pepper, minced garlic, and lemon zest.
3. Trim asparagus spears and toss with olive oil, salt, and pepper.

4. Place a few asparagus spears on top of each salmon fillet and wrap tightly.
5. Arrange salmon and asparagus bundles on the prepared baking sheet.
6. Bake in the oven until salmon is cooked through and asparagus is tender.
7. Serve hot with lemon wedges.

Prep Time: 10 minutes

Cook Time: 20 minutes

Total Time: 30 minutes

Customization: Use other fish fillets like cod or halibut, and add a sprinkle of dried herbs like dill or thyme.

Cucumber and Dill Salad with Smoked Salmon

Ingredients:

- Cucumber
- Smoked salmon
- Greek yogurt
- Fresh dill
- Lemon juice
- Olive oil
- Salt and pepper

Instructions:

1. Thinly slice cucumber and place in a bowl.
2. Flake smoked salmon and add to the bowl.
3. In a separate bowl, mix Greek yogurt, chopped fresh dill, lemon juice, olive oil, salt, and pepper to make the dressing.
4. Pour the dressing over the cucumber and smoked salmon, and toss to coat.
5. Serve chilled as a refreshing salad.

Prep Time: 10 minutes

Total Time: 10 minutes

Customization: Add diced red onion or capers for extra flavor.

Bunless Burger with Grilled Vegetables

Ingredients:

- Ground beef (or turkey)
- Lettuce leaves
- Tomato
- Red onion
- Pickles
- Mustard
- Mayonnaise
- Olive oil
- Salt and pepper

Instructions:

1. Season ground beef with salt and pepper, then shape into patties.

2. Grill or pan-sear the burger patties until cooked to your liking.
3. Slice tomato and red onion, and wash lettuce leaves.
4. Assemble burgers by wrapping the cooked patties in lettuce leaves and topping with sliced tomato, red onion, pickles, mustard, and mayonnaise.
5. Serve with grilled vegetables on the side.

Prep Time: 10 minutes

Cook Time: 10 minutes

Total Time: 20 minutes

Customization: Use portobello mushrooms or eggplant slices instead of burger patties for a vegetarian option.

Caprese Salad with Balsamic Reduction

Ingredients:

- Fresh mozzarella cheese
- Tomatoes
- Fresh basil
- Balsamic vinegar
- Olive oil
- Salt and pepper

Instructions:

1. Slice fresh mozzarella cheese and tomatoes into rounds.

2. Arrange alternating slices of mozzarella cheese, tomato, and fresh basil leaves on a plate.
3. Drizzle with balsamic vinegar and olive oil.
4. Season with salt and pepper to taste.

Prep Time: 10 minutes

Total Time: 10 minutes

Customization: Add sliced avocado or prosciutto for extra richness and flavor.

Dinner Recipes

Grilled Steak with Herb Butter

Ingredients:

- Steak (such as ribeye, sirloin)
- Butter
- Fresh herbs (such as parsley, thyme, rosemary)
- Garlic
- Salt and pepper

Instructions:

1. Season steak with salt and pepper.

2. Grill steak to desired doneness.
3. Meanwhile, mix softened butter with chopped herbs and minced garlic.
4. Place a dollop of herb butter on top of the grilled steak before serving.

Prep Time: 10 minutes

Cook Time: 10-15 minutes

Total Time: 20-25 minutes

Customization: Use different herb combinations for the butter, such as cilantro and lime for a Tex-Mex twist.

Lemon and Herb Roasted Chicken

Ingredients:

- Chicken pieces (such as thighs, drumsticks)
- Lemon
- Fresh herbs (such as thyme, rosemary)
- Garlic
- Olive oil
- Salt and pepper

Instructions:

1. Preheat oven and place chicken pieces in a baking dish.
2. Squeeze lemon juice over the chicken and season with salt and pepper.
3. Scatter fresh herbs and minced garlic over the chicken.
4. Drizzle with olive oil.
5. Roast in the oven until the chicken is cooked through and golden brown.

Prep Time: 10 minutes

Cook Time: 40-45 minutes

Total Time: 50-55 minutes

Customization: Add sliced onions or potatoes to the baking dish for extra flavor and texture.

Pork Tenderloin with Mustard Sauce

Ingredients:

- Pork tenderloin
- Dijon mustard
- Honey (or sugar-free sweetener for keto)
- Garlic
- Chicken broth
- Olive oil
- Salt and pepper

Instructions:

1. Season pork tenderloin with salt and pepper.
2. Sear pork tenderloin in a skillet until browned on all sides.
3. In the same skillet, mix Dijon mustard, honey, minced garlic, and chicken broth.

4. Simmer until the sauce thickens.
5. Slice pork tenderloin and serve with mustard sauce drizzled on top.

Prep Time: 10 minutes

Cook Time: 20-25 minutes

Total Time: 30-35 minutes

Customization: Use whole grain mustard for added texture and tanginess.

Seared Tuna Steaks with Olive Tapenade

Ingredients:

- Tuna steaks
- Olives (such as Kalamata or green)
- Capers
- Garlic
- Lemon juice
- Olive oil
- Salt and pepper

Instructions:

1. Season tuna steaks with salt and pepper.
2. Sear tuna steaks in a hot skillet or grill until browned on both sides but still pink in the center.
3. Meanwhile, make olive tapenade by blending olives, capers, minced garlic, lemon juice, and olive oil until chunky.
4. Serve seared tuna steaks with a dollop of olive tapenade on top.

Prep Time: 10 minutes

Cook Time: 5 minutes

Total Time: 15 minutes

Customization: Add chopped sun-dried tomatoes or anchovies to the olive tapenade for extra depth of flavor.

Cauliflower Steak with Walnut Pesto

Ingredients:

- Cauliflower
- Walnuts
- Basil
- Parmesan cheese
- Garlic
- Lemon juice
- Olive oil
- Salt and pepper

Instructions:

1. Slice cauliflower into thick "steaks."
2. Roast cauliflower steaks in the oven until tender and golden brown.
3. Meanwhile, make walnut pesto by blending walnuts, basil, grated Parmesan cheese, minced garlic, lemon juice, and olive oil until smooth.

4. Serve roasted cauliflower steaks with a generous spoonful of walnut pesto on top.

Prep Time: 10 minutes

Cook Time: 25-30 minutes

Total Time: 35-40 minutes

Customization: Add a pinch of red pepper flakes for a hint of heat in the pesto.

Baked Cod with Olives and Tomatoes

Ingredients:

- Cod fillets
- Cherry tomatoes
- Olives (such as Kalamata or black)
- Garlic
- Olive oil
- Lemon
- Fresh parsley
- Salt and pepper

Instructions:

1. Preheat oven and place cod fillets in a baking dish.
2. Scatter halved cherry tomatoes and pitted olives around the cod.
3. Drizzle with olive oil and sprinkle minced garlic over the top.

4. Squeeze lemon juice over the fish and season with salt and pepper.
5. Bake in the oven until the fish is opaque and flakes easily with a fork.
6. Garnish with chopped fresh parsley before serving.

Prep Time: 10 minutes

Cook Time: 15-20 minutes

Total Time: 25-30 minutes

Customization: Add sliced bell peppers or onions for extra flavor and color.

Lamb Chops with Mint Pesto

Ingredients:

- Lamb chops
- Mint leaves
- Pine nuts
- Parmesan cheese
- Garlic
- Lemon juice
- Olive oil
- Salt and pepper

Instructions:

1. Season lamb chops with salt and pepper.
2. Grill or pan-sear lamb chops until cooked to your liking.
3. Meanwhile, make mint pesto by blending mint leaves, toasted

pine nuts, grated Parmesan cheese, minced garlic, lemon juice, and olive oil until smooth.

4. Serve grilled lamb chops with a dollop of mint pesto on top.

Prep Time: 10 minutes

Cook Time: 10-15 minutes

Total Time: 20-25 minutes

Customization: Add a pinch of cumin or coriander to the mint pesto for an extra layer of flavor.

Turkey Meatballs in Marinara Sauce

Ingredients:

- Ground turkey
- Bread crumbs (or almond flour for keto)
- Egg
- Garlic
- Parmesan cheese
- Italian seasoning
- Tomato sauce
- Olive oil
- Salt and pepper

Instructions:

1. Preheat oven and line a baking sheet with parchment paper.
2. Mix ground turkey, bread crumbs, beaten egg, minced garlic, grated Parmesan cheese, and Italian seasoning in a bowl until well combined.
3. Shape mixture into meatballs and place them on the prepared baking sheet.
4. Bake in the oven until meatballs are cooked through and golden brown.
5. Meanwhile, heat tomato sauce in a saucepan.
6. Serve turkey meatballs with marinara sauce spooned over the top.

Prep Time: 15 minutes

Cook Time: 20-25 minutes

Total Time: 35-40 minutes

Customization: Use ground beef or chicken instead of turkey, and add chopped fresh herbs like parsley or basil to the meatball mixture for extra flavor.

Spicy Grilled Shrimp

Ingredients:

- Shrimp
- Chili powder
- Paprika
- Garlic powder
- Olive oil
- Lime juice
- Salt and pepper

Instructions:

1. Season shrimp with chili powder, paprika, garlic powder, olive oil, lime juice, salt, and pepper.
2. Thread shrimp onto skewers and grill until pink and slightly charred.
3. Serve hot as an appetizer or main dish.

Prep Time: 10 minutes

Cook Time: 5 minutes

Total Time: 15 minutes

Customization: Add cayenne pepper or hot sauce for extra heat, or serve with a side of creamy avocado sauce for dipping.

Garlic Butter Mushrooms

Ingredients:

- Mushrooms
- Butter
- Garlic
- Fresh parsley
- Lemon juice
- Salt and pepper

Instructions:

1. Clean mushrooms and slice them if they are large.
2. Melt butter in a skillet over medium heat.
3. Add minced garlic to the skillet and cook until fragrant.

4. Add mushrooms to the skillet and sauté until golden brown and tender.
5. Season with salt, pepper, and chopped fresh parsley.
6. Finish with a squeeze of lemon juice before serving.

Prep Time: 10 minutes

Cook Time: 10 minutes

Total Time: 20 minutes

Customization: Add white wine or balsamic vinegar for extra flavor, or sprinkle with grated Parmesan cheese before serving.

Roasted Duck with Orange Sauce

Ingredients:

- Duck breasts
- Oranges
- Honey
- Soy sauce
- Garlic
- Ginger
- Olive oil
- Salt and pepper

Instructions:

1. Preheat oven and score the skin of duck breasts.
2. Season duck breasts with salt and pepper.

3. Roast duck breasts in the oven until skin is crispy and meat is cooked to your liking.
4. Meanwhile, make orange sauce by simmering orange juice, honey, soy sauce, minced garlic, and grated ginger until thickened.
5. Serve roasted duck breasts with orange sauce drizzled on top.

Prep Time: 10 minutes

Cook Time: 30-40 minutes

Total Time: 40-50 minutes

Customization: Add a splash of Grand Marnier or brandy to the orange sauce for an extra depth of flavor.

Herb-Crusted Rack of Lamb

Ingredients:

- Rack of lamb
- Fresh herbs (such as rosemary, thyme)
- Garlic
- Dijon mustard
- Bread crumbs (or almond flour for keto)
- Olive oil
- Salt and pepper

Instructions:

1. Preheat oven and season rack of lamb with salt and pepper.

2. Mix chopped fresh herbs, minced garlic, Dijon mustard, bread crumbs, and olive oil in a bowl to form a paste.
3. Press herb mixture onto the meaty side of the rack of lamb.
4. Roast in the oven until the crust is golden brown and the lamb is cooked to your liking.
5. Let the lamb rest before slicing and serving.

Prep Time: 15 minutes

Cook Time: 25-30 minutes

Total Time: 40-45 minutes

Customization: Use a mixture of different herbs like parsley and mint for the crust.

Grilled Mahi Mahi with Mango Salsa

Ingredients:

- Mahi mahi fillets
- Mango
- Red bell pepper
- Red onion
- Cilantro
- Lime juice
- Olive oil
- Salt and pepper

Instructions:

1. Season mahimahi fillets with salt, pepper, and a drizzle of olive oil.
2. Grill mahimahi fillets until cooked through and flaky.
3. Meanwhile, make mango salsa by combining diced mango, diced red bell pepper, diced red onion, chopped cilantro, lime juice, olive oil, salt, and pepper in a bowl.
4. Serve grilled mahimahi fillets with mango salsa spooned on top.

Prep Time: 15 minutes

Cook Time: 10 minutes

Total Time: 25 minutes

Customization: Add diced jalapeño for a spicy kick in the mango salsa.

Roast Beef with Creamy Horseradish Sauce

Ingredients:

- Beef roast (such as sirloin or ribeye)
- Horseradish
- Sour cream (or Greek yogurt for a lighter option)
- Dijon mustard
- Garlic
- Olive oil
- Salt and pepper

Instructions:

1. Preheat oven and season beef roast with salt and pepper.
2. Roast beef in the oven until cooked to your desired doneness.
3. Meanwhile, make creamy horseradish sauce by mixing horseradish, sour cream, Dijon mustard, minced garlic, olive oil, salt, and pepper in a bowl.
4. Let the beef roast rest before slicing thinly.
5. Serve roast beef slices with creamy horseradish sauce on the side.

Prep Time: 15 minutes

Cook Time: Variable (depends on the size of the roast)

Total Time: Variable

Customization: Add a splash of Worcestershire sauce or a pinch of sugar to balance the flavors in the horseradish sauce.

Keto Jambalaya

Ingredients:

- Cauliflower rice
- Shrimp
- Andouille sausage
- Chicken thighs
- Bell peppers

- Celery
- Onion
- Garlic
- Diced tomatoes
- Cajun seasoning
- Chicken broth
- Olive oil
- Salt and pepper

Instructions:

1. Heat olive oil in a large skillet or Dutch oven over medium heat.
2. Add diced onion, celery, and bell peppers to the skillet and cook until softened.
3. Stir in minced garlic and Cajun seasoning, and cook until fragrant.
4. Add diced chicken thighs and sliced Andouille sausage to the skillet and cook until browned.
5. Stir in cauliflower rice, diced tomatoes, and chicken broth.
6. Simmer until the cauliflower rice is tender and the flavors have melded together.
7. Add shrimp to the skillet and cook until pink and cooked through.
8. Season with salt and pepper to taste before serving.

Prep Time: 20 minutes

Cook Time: 25-30 minutes

Total Time: 45-50 minutes

Customization: Add diced ham or crawfish for a traditional jambalaya flavor, or garnish with chopped green onions and parsley before serving.

Snacks Recipes

Celery Sticks with Almond Butter

Ingredients:

- Celery sticks
- Almond butter

Instructions:

Wash and cut celery stalks into sticks.
Spread almond butter on each celery stick.

Prep Time: 5 minutes

Total Time: 5 minutes

Customization: Substitute almond butter with other nut or seed butter like peanut butter or sunflower seed butter.

Cheese Crisps

Ingredients:

- Cheese slices (such as cheddar or parmesan)

Instructions:

- Preheat oven and line a baking sheet with parchment paper.

- Cut cheese slices into smaller squares or rectangles.
- Place cheese slices on the baking sheet with space in between.
- Bake in the oven until the edges are golden brown and crispy.
- Let cool before serving.

Prep Time: 5 minutes

Cook Time: 5-7 minutes

Total Time: 10-12 minutes

Customization: Add herbs or spices like garlic powder or smoked paprika for extra flavor.

Boiled Eggs with Paprika

Ingredients:

- Eggs
- Paprika
- Salt and pepper

Instructions:

1. Boil eggs in water until cooked to your desired doneness.
2. Peel the eggs and cut them in half lengthwise.
3. Sprinkle paprika, salt, and pepper over the boiled eggs.

Prep Time: 2 minutes

Cook Time: 10-12 minutes

Total Time: 12-14 minutes

Customization: Replace paprika with chili powder or cayenne pepper for a spicy kick.

Avocado Chocolate Mousse

Ingredients:

- Avocado
- Cocoa powder
- Honey (or sweetener of choice)
- Vanilla extract

Instructions:

1. Scoop avocado flesh into a blender or food processor.
2. Add cocoa powder, honey, and vanilla extract.
3. Blend until smooth and creamy.
4. Chill in the refrigerator before serving.

Prep Time: 5 minutes

Total Time: 5 minutes

Customization: Add a pinch of sea salt or cinnamon for extra flavor dimension.

Kale Chips

Ingredients:

- Kale leaves
- Olive oil
- Salt

Instructions:

1. Preheat oven and line a baking sheet with parchment paper.
2. Remove stems from kale leaves and tear into bite-sized pieces.
3. Toss kale pieces with olive oil and spread them on the baking sheet.
4. Sprinkle with salt.
5. Bake in the oven until crispy, about 10-15 minutes.

Prep Time: 10 minutes

Cook Time: 10-15 minutes

Total Time: 20-25 minutes

Customization: Sprinkle with grated Parmesan cheese or nutritional yeast for a cheesy flavor.

Beef Jerky

Ingredients:

- Beef (such as flank steak or sirloin)
- Soy sauce (or coconut aminos for gluten-free)
- Worcestershire sauce
- Liquid smoke
- Garlic powder
- Onion powder
- Black pepper

Instructions:

1. Slice beef thinly against the grain.
2. Mix soy sauce, Worcestershire sauce, liquid smoke, garlic powder, onion powder, and black pepper in a bowl to make a marinade.
3. Marinate beef slices in the mixture for several hours or overnight.
4. Dehydrate beef slices in a food dehydrator or oven until dry and chewy.

Prep Time: 15 minutes (plus marinating time)

Cook Time: Variable (depends on the drying method)

Total Time: Variable

Customization: Add chili flakes or hot sauce for a spicy version.

Stuffed Jalapeños with Cream Cheese

Ingredients:

- Jalapeños
- Cream cheese
- Bacon (optional)

Instructions:

1. Cut jalapeños in half lengthwise and remove seeds.
2. Fill each jalapeño half with cream cheese.
3. Wrap with bacon if desired.

4. Bake in the oven until jalapeños are softened and bacon is crispy.

Prep Time: 10 minutes

Cook Time: 15-20 minutes

Total Time: 25-30 minutes

Customization: Mix chopped herbs or shredded cheese into the cream cheese for added flavor.

Cucumber Slices with Hummus

Ingredients:

- Cucumber
- Hummus

Instructions:

1. Slice cucumber into rounds or sticks.
2. Serve with hummus for dipping.

Prep Time: 5 minutes

Total Time: 5 minutes

Customization: Use flavored hummus such as roasted red pepper or garlic for variety.

Macadamia Nuts

Ingredients:

- Macadamia nuts

Instructions:

1. Enjoy macadamia nuts as they are, or roast them in the oven for extra flavor.

Prep Time: 1 minute

Total Time: 1 minute (or longer if roasting)

Customization: Mix with other nuts like almonds or cashews for a mixed nut snack.

Caprese Skewers with Cherry Tomatoes and Mozzarella

Ingredients:

- Cherry tomatoes
- Fresh mozzarella balls (or cubed mozzarella cheese)
- Fresh basil leaves
- Balsamic glaze (optional)
- Olive oil (optional)
- Salt and pepper

Instructions:

1. Thread cherry tomatoes, mozzarella balls, and basil leaves onto skewers.
2. Drizzle with balsamic glaze and olive oil, if desired.
3. Season with salt and pepper to taste.

Prep Time: 10 minutes

Total Time: 10 minutes

Customization: Add a slice of prosciutto or grilled chicken to each skewer for extra protein.

4-Week Meal Plan
Week 1: Kickstarting Your Metabolism

Day	Breakfast	Lunch	Dinner	Snacks
Monday	Banana Oat Pancakes	Chicken Caesar Salad	Grilled Steak with Herb Butter	Celery Sticks with Almond Butter
Tuesday	Blueberry Muffins with Honey	Zucchini Noodle Salad with Pesto	Lemon and Herb Roasted Chicken	Cheese Crisps
Wednesday	Maple and Brown Sugar Oatmeal	Tuna Salad Stuffed Avocados	Cauliflower Steak with Walnut Pesto	Boiled Eggs with Paprika
Thursday	Sweet Potato and Black Bean Breakfast Burritos	Stuffed Bell Peppers with Ground Turkey	Seared Tuna Steaks with Olive Tapenade	Avocado Chocolate Mousse
Friday	Apple Cinnamon French Toast	Broccoli and Stilton Soup	Baked Cod with Olives and Tomatoes	Kale Chips
Saturday	Quinoa and Fruit Breakfast Bowl	Eggplant and Tomato Stacks with Feta Cheese	Lamb Chops with Mint Pesto	Beef Jerky
Sunday	Cranberry Almond Granola	Beef and Vegetable Stir Fry	Turkey Meatballs in Marinara Sauce	Stuffed Jalapeños with Cream Cheese

Week 2: Deepening the Impact

Day	Breakfast	Lunch	Dinner	Snacks
Monday	Pumpkin Spice Waffles	Mediterranean Couscous Salad	Pork Tenderloin with Mustard Sauce	Cucumber Slices with Hummus
Tuesday	Caramelized Pear and Brie Crepes	Spaghetti with Sun-dried Tomato Pesto	Spicy Grilled Shrimp	Macadamia Nuts
Wednesday	Bagel with Cream Cheese and Smoked Salmon	Pasta Primavera with Spring Vegetables	Garlic Butter Mushrooms	Stuffed Jalapeños with Cream Cheese
Thursday	Cherry and Almond Porridge	Sweet Corn and Zucchini Pie	Roasted Duck with Orange Sauce	Celery Sticks with Almond Butter
Friday	Raspberry Yogurt Parfait	Grilled Vegetable and Hummus Tart	Herb-Crusted Rack of Lamb	Cheese Crisps
Saturday	Energy Balls with Oats and Dates	Asian Noodle Salad with Peanut Dressing	Grilled Mahi Mahi with Mango Salsa	Boiled Eggs with Paprika
Sunday	Homemade Banana Bread	Roasted Beet and Citrus Salad	Roast Beef with Creamy Horseradish Sauce	Avocado Chocolate Mousse

Week 3: The Metabolic Boost

Day	Breakfast	Lunch	Dinner	Snacks
Monday	Avocado and Egg Breakfast Bowl	Chicken Lettuce Wraps	Potato Gnocchi with Tomato Basil Sauce	Kale Chips
Tuesday	Spinach and Mushroom Omelette	Salmon and Asparagus Bundles	Creamy Polenta with Roasted Mushrooms	Cheese Crisps
Wednesday	Greek Yogurt with Nuts and Seeds	Cucumber and Dill Salad with Smoked Salmon	Vegetable Paella	Boiled Eggs with Paprika
Thursday	Smoked Salmon and Cream Cheese Roll-Ups	Caprese Salad with Balsamic Reduction	Lentil and Sweet Potato Shepherd's Pie	Macadamia Nuts
Friday	Cauliflower Hash Browns	Bunless Burger with Grilled Vegetables	Stuffed Acorn Squash with Quinoa and Cranberries	Celery Sticks with Almond Butter
Saturday	Almond Flour Pancakes	Moroccan Vegetable Tagine	Chickpea and Spinach Curry	Stuffed Jalapeños with Cream Cheese
Sunday	Coconut and Chia Seed Pudding	Eggplant Parmesan	Stuffed Peppers with Rice and Beans	Avocado Chocolate Mousse

Week 4: The Home Stretch

Day	Breakfast	Lunch	Dinner	Snacks
Monday	Turkey and Spinach Scrambled Eggs	Zucchini and Tomato Tart	Spaghetti with Sun-dried Tomato Pesto	Cheese Crisps
Tuesday	Bacon and Egg Muffins	Chicken Caesar Salad (no croutons)	Vegetable Paella	Macadamia Nuts
Wednesday	Cheese and Herb Frittata	Salmon and Asparagus Bundles	Teriyaki Tofu with Sticky Rice	Stuffed Jalapeños with Cream Cheese
Thursday	Avocado and Egg Breakfast Bowl	Tuna Salad Stuffed Avocados	Stuffed Bell Peppers with Ground Turkey	Celery Sticks with Almond Butter
Friday	Protein Smoothie with Avocado and Cocoa	Broccoli and Stilton Soup	Grilled Steak with Herb Butter	Kale Chips
Saturday	Quinoa and Fruit Breakfast Bowl	Beef and Vegetable Stir Fry	Cauliflower Steak with Walnut Pesto	Avocado Chocolate Mousse
Sunday	Spinach and Mushroom Omelette	Chicken Lettuce Wraps	Roast Beef with Creamy Horseradish Sauce	Boiled Eggs with Paprika

This 4-week meal plan incorporates a variety of delicious and nutritious recipes while alternating between high carb and low carb days, following the principles of carb cycling.

Conclusion

As we conclude our journey through the Carb Cycling Cookbook, we hope you feel empowered with the knowledge and tools necessary to achieve sustainable weight loss and effortless slimming. Carb cycling is more than just a diet; it's a lifestyle that can transform not only your body but also your relationship with food and your overall well-being.

Throughout this guide, we've explored the science behind carb cycling, the practical steps to implement it into your daily life, and an array of delicious recipes to keep you satisfied along the way. By understanding the role of macros, setting realistic goals, and embracing a balanced approach to nutrition, you have the power to achieve your fitness goals and maintain them for the long term.

Remember, success with carb cycling is not about perfection but consistency. Embrace the journey, celebrate your victories, and learn from your setbacks. Whether you're embarking on this path for the first time or seeking a fresh approach to reignite your progress, know that you have the support and resources you need to succeed.

As you continue your carb cycling journey, may you discover newfound energy, confidence, and joy in nourishing your body and achieving your goals. Here's to a healthier, happier you – one delicious meal and balanced choice at a time.

Must Read!!!

Thank you for choosing to explore my book! Your support means the world to me. As a valued reader, your review holds immense significance. Your insights not only guide potential readers but also contribute to shaping the ongoing journey of this book. Your thoughts help in fostering a community of engaged readers, making the experience richer for everyone.

How You Can Share Your Review?

Sharing your review on Amazon allows others to benefit from your perspective, aiding them in their decision-making process.

To post your review, simply visit the Amazon page where you discovered my book, head to the 'Customer Reviews' section, and click on 'Write a customer review' to share your invaluable feedback.

Alternatively, you can effortlessly access the review section by scanning the QR code below with your smartphone. Thank you once again for your support and for considering sharing your thoughts with us.